Edited by
DORA BLACK, JEAN HARRIS-HENDRIKS,
STEPHEN WOLKIND

with contributions from
RICHARD WHITE　　ULOMEW'S

Foreword
LADY J　　　　UTLER-SLOSS

Child Psychiatry
and the Law

Third Edition

GASKELL

© The Royal College of Psychiatrists 1989, 1991, 1998

First published 1989
Second edition 1991
Third edition 1998

British Library Cataloguing-in-Publication Data
A catalogue record for this book is available from
the British Library.

ISBN 1-901242-14-5 3rd edn
(ISBN 0-902241-41-9 2nd edn,
ISBN 0-902241-31-1 1st edn)

Gaskell is an imprint of the Royal College of Psychiatrists,
17 Belgrave Square, London SW1X 8PG

Distributed in North America
by American Psychiatric Press, Inc.
ISBN 0-88048-584-1

The views presented in this book do not necessarily reflect
those of the Royal College of Psychiatrists, and the publishers
are not responsible for any error of omission or fact.

The Royal College of Psychiatrists is a registered charity (no. 228636).

Printed by Bell & Bain Ltd, Thornliebank, Glasgow.

Contents

List of contributors

Robin Benians, Former Consultant Psychiatrist, Ealing Child Guidance Service and Barnardos

Arnon Bentovim, Honorary Consultant Child Psychiatrist, Hospital for Sick Children, Great Ormond Street and the Tavistock Clinic. Honorary Senior Lecturer, Institute of Child Health, London

Ian Berg, Former Consultant in Child and Adolescent Psychiatry, Leeds General Infirmary. Senior Clinical Lecturer, University of Leeds

Dora Black, Honorary Consultant Child and Adolescent Psychiatrist, Traumatic Stress Clinic, Camden and Islington Community Services NHS Trust. Honorary Consultant, Royal Free Hospital, Great Ormond Street Hospital for Children and Tavistock Clinic, London. Honorary Senior Lecturer, Royal Free Hospital School of Medicine and University College, London

David Cottrell, Professor of Child and Adolescent Psychiatry, School of Medicine, University of Leeds

Ann Gath, Consultant Developmental Psychiatrist, Suffolk

Martyn Gay, Former Consultant Child and Adolescent Psychiatrist, Royal Hospital for Sick Children, Bristol

Alyson Hall, Consultant Child and Adolescent Psychiatrist, Tower Hamlets Healthcare Trust. Honorary Senior Lecturer, London Hospital Medical College

Peter Harris, Official Solicitor to the Supreme Court

Jean Harris-Hendriks, Consultant Child and Adolescent Psychiatrist, Traumatic Stress Clinic, Camden and Islington Community Services NHS Trust. Honorary Senior Lecturer, Royal Free Hospital School of Medicine and University College, London

Peter Hill, Professor of Child Mental Health and Consultant in Child and Adolescent Psychiatry, St George's Hospital Medical School, University of London

Mary Lindsay, Former Consultant Child and Adolescent Psychiatrist, Buckinghamshire

Alan McClelland, Former Consultant Child and Adolescent Psychiatrist, St George's Hospital, London (died July 1998)

Carol Sheldrick, Consultant Forensic Psychiatrist, Children's and Adolescents' Department, Maudsley Hospital, London

Margaret J. Thompson, Consultant Child and Adolescent Psychiatrist, Southampton Community Health Services

Judith Trowell, Consultant Child and Adolescent Psychiatrist, Tavistock Clinic. Consultant and Honorary, Senior Lecturer, Royal Free Hospital, London. Chairperson, Young Minds, National Association for Child and Family Mental Health

Guinevere Tufnell, Consultant Psychiatrist, Child and Family Consultation Service, Forest Healthcare Trust, London

Kirk Weir, Consultant Psychiatrist, Institute of Family Therapy, Ipswich, Suffolk

Richard White, Partner, White and Sherwin, Solicitors, Croydon

Stephen Wolkind, Emeritus Consultant Psychiatrist, Maudsley Hospital, London

Harry Zeitlin, Professor of Child and Adolescent Psychiatry, University College, London

Foreword

LADY JUSTICE BUTLER-SLOSS

Recent events have underlined the importance of effective preparation of evidence in proceedings relating to children. Clearly presented written reports setting out the facts, the conclusions and reasons are important for all professionals involved in court proceedings of any kind. There is an added dimension with children, whose welfare is at the heart of the proceedings before the court.

The medical profession and particularly the child psychiatrists have an increasingly crucial role to play in cases involving the welfare of children, both in the provision of written reports and in frequently being required to give oral evidence in addition. The information provided by the child psychiatrist may be the deciding factor, for instance, in removing the child from the family or risking the return of the child to the family. The method of presentation of a report may have a marked effect upon its usefulness to the court asked to rely on it, and the ability to present the facts succinctly and clearly, to explain the reasons for conclusions which can be summarised and clearly understood by laymen therefore assumes great importance. To be able to think clearly about a child's problems and to explain them in simple language to a court by way of oral evidence is of equal importance. Those engaged in this demanding work and called as experts may not be expert witnesses. An understanding of the requirements of the particular court and of the proceedings for which the expertise of the child psychiatrist is needed makes the task of the expert easier and his efforts more valuable.

This book, with its careful and detailed advice to its readers as to the compilation of reports and presentation of the relevant material, fills a large gap in a most helpful and constructive manner. The combined experience of the authors in the medico-legal field gives the book great authority, and the practical instruction, together with the check-lists, will, I am sure, be invaluable both to the practitioner new to medico-legal work and also to those more experienced, who will find much of use in its pages.

The advice extends beyond the courts, to the agencies who may need the help of child psychiatrists, and the book gives a valuable and simple insight into the complex jungle of the present child care legislation. The second part of this volume gives very useful specimen reports.

This is not only a most useful guide for child psychiatrists, all of whom from time to time may be involved in child care or matrimonial child disputes, but also for a wider audience of readers who may from this book find it easier to understand the role of the child psychiatrist.

Preface to the third edition

The Children Act 1989, England and Wales, implemented in October 1991, together with complementary changes in juvenile justice, adoption and education law, have necessitated a third edition. Concepts such as 'significant harm', 'emergency protection order', 'residence' and 'contact' orders have been established and new case law achieved. Chapter 13, section II has been rewritten by Richard White who has also supplied a glossary and an overview of key legal decisions and advice. Recent research and literature reviews are referenced and the recommended reading list has been updated.

DB, JHH, SW, 1998

Introduction

DORA BLACK, JEAN HARRIS-HENDRIKS AND STEPHEN WOLKIND

Until the 1970s, child and adolescent psychiatry was one of the most private and even secretive of medical specialities. The role of the practitioner was to see the patient alone, and slowly help the child towards mental health. The essence of this work was the total confidentiality of the relationship between child and psychiatrist. Although parents were interviewed, information proffered by the patient was treated as sacrosanct and would be passed on neither to parents nor to other professionals. Child and adolescent psychiatrists needed rarely to expose their techniques to the scrutiny of colleagues nor to defend their views in public.

This has now changed dramatically, partly because of new trends in clinical practice. Family therapy with its vigorous approach has made customary the one-way screen and video recorder. Child and adolescent psychiatrists will now readily demonstrate, to their colleagues, the way they work. The increase in consultative work, which may take up to 30% of the time of many practitioners, involves sharing one's views with multi-disciplinary teams.

Perhaps the greatest change, however, has arisen out of the amount of medico-legal work which is now being carried out by child and adolescent psychiatrists. Reports describing a child's psychological functioning will be read by large numbers of people and psychiatrists will have to defend their opinions in front of the legal profession, social workers and family members. There are no adequate data but throughout the United Kingdom most child and adolescent psychiatrists do find that an increased amount of their time involves the preparation of court reports and attendance at courts of law.

A number of factors have contributed to this trend. The first lies within the nature of child and adolescent psychiatry itself. Initially a very personal speciality with success possibly depending on the skill of a particular worker, it has evolved into one with a strong research tradition and a growing database.

In parallel with other fields of medicine, child and adolescent psychiatrists can now speak in terms of probabilities in outcome. Relevant findings have been published in scientifically sound and well-written books and have been read by social workers and lawyers. The child and adolescent psychiatrist is seen as the expert who can state how one child's needs can be interpreted against this background (see Wolkind, 1994). The second major factor lies outside child and adolescent psychiatry and in society's views of the rights of children. Just as society became shocked in the 1960s by a growing awareness of physical abuse, so in the 1980s and 1990s it has been affected by the publicity given to emotional and sexual abuse and the effects upon children of war, civil conflict and man-made and natural disasters. The child and adolescent psychiatrist has joined the paediatrician and radiologist as an important diagnostician. Thus we now have to give opinions as to whether a child's behaviour is such that emotional development and the capacity to form attachments are being impaired and whether that impairment may be due to abuse, neglect or other forms of psychological trauma. We then need to advise on what course of action might be in the child's best interests. The greater recognition of the child's rights has led to children being independently represented in courts and the wide use of guardians ad litem. Many guardians, who often work in isolation, have been particularly keen to have the help of child and adolescent psychiatrists. There is a requirement also for improved evaluation of the needs of children and their increased representation in private law hearings, where conflicts between adults, as in divorce, do not involve the state but are profoundly upsetting to the children caught up in them.

Doctors have always had an uneasy relationship with the legal profession. It is not surprising that many child and adolescent psychiatrists are reluctant to have any dealing with this sort of work. It goes against all our traditions of confidentiality. It may also represent a threat to the autonomy and authority of the practitioner. No doctor likes to be criticised or even to be exposed to ridicule, albeit in the closed courts where hearings concerning children are held. Nevertheless, the work has increased. Most psychiatrists have been pleasantly surprised by the courtesy with which all parties have dealt with them. If it is plain that the aim of the psychiatrist is to provide evidence which will attempt to help the child, irrespective of who has requested the psychiatric opinion, and that dogmatic views are not held, all sides do seem to listen to our views with respect. They might not accept them. Matters other than purely psychiatric ones, rightly, will influence the decision of a court, but in general, our views will be considered seriously. An appearance in court can be unpleasant and even harrowing. For example, it is never pleasant to give an opinion suggesting that a mentally ill parent should be deprived of a child, knowing that that parent is in court listening and suffering as one speaks. Against this, however, is the knowledge that a well-formulated argument can help release a child to a new, safer life, or be started on a long-overdue rehabilitation programme. Sometimes legal intervention can be more effective than many years of treatment, although usually we will realise there is no perfect answer and at best we can hope to obtain 'the least detrimental' solution (Goldstein *et al*, 1980*a*).

With familiarity, the terrors of court tend to recede, but an alternative menace can arise. There is often an excitement about the adversarial proceedings with lawyers lined up on each side. It can be easy for medical specialists to be seduced into partisan support of those who have asked them to provide evidence. There is nothing less edifying than having two psychiatrists giving different opinions rather than attempting constructively to examine the reasons for any difference in emphasis in their recommendations. In fact, a requirement from the Family Division of the Supreme Court is that experts should consult prior to a hearing and the judge be supplied with a written account of areas of agreement and disagreement.

This book developed out of a series of discussions held by the contributors – a group of child and adolescent psychiatrists active in medico-legal work. Its prime aim is to help trainees and newly appointed consultant child and adolescent psychiatrists prepare themselves for work as professional and expert witnesses. It is also hoped that it will prove useful to those in related professions, such as psychology, paediatrics and social work, who may be called upon to do similar tasks. In addition, it should demonstrate to lawyers, judges, guardians ad litem and court welfare officers what they might reasonably expect from a child and adolescent psychiatrist, and what his or her contribution could be in dealing with the future of a child. Although the legal aspects of this book apply only to England and Wales, we would hope that the psychiatric principles would be relevant within any jurisdiction. (It is essential that child and adolescent psychiatrists are abreast of the law concerning children.)

Doctors may be involved professionally with legal matters in criminal or civil proceedings. As any citizen, they may be called as a 'witness to fact', giving evidence on an incident they have witnessed, or as a 'professional witness', for example giving evidence relating to one of their own patients. They may be called also as an 'expert witness', by one of the parties in a dispute, or by the court. They may be asked to give an expert opinion on someone who is not their patient, using specialised knowledge and experience.

The first five chapters deal with general issues, referral and assessment, writing a report and presenting evidence, and discuss the roles of local and outside experts, and issues of confidentiality. The word *forensic*, which derives from *forum*, refers to all legal work which may bring medical practitioners into the public domain including criminal law. Chapter 2 discusses the role of psychiatrists in the juvenile justice system. The chapter on report writing has been rewritten in the light of research by Guinevere Tufnell and David Cottrell formulated as advice to expert witnesses by Peter Harris, Official Solicitor to the Supreme Court, reproduced with his permission. Chapters 6 to 12 deal with specific issues relating to delinquency, compensation claims, educational issues, child abuse and child care. For child and adolescent psychiatry it is the latter two areas of work which have expanded recently and we have therefore devoted more space to issues about residence and contact, assessing parenting capacity, adoption issues and sexual abuse. Ann Gath has contributed a note on the assessment of parents with learning disability, Alyson Hall has reviewed the literature on contact and Peter Hill has rewritten Chapter 10 on compensation claims.

At the end of relevant chapters will be found a check-list which, we hope, will serve as an *aide-mémoire* when speaking to a referrer, making a report or attending a court.

Chapter 11, Education, and Chapter 12, Juvenile justice, take account of current law.

Chapter 13 discusses child law and contains a revised section by Richard White, a solicitor who specialises in, and has written extensively about, child care legal practice, outlining the relevant legal framework and recent decisions and guidance which affect the presentation of expert evidence.

The Children Act 1989, discussed in Chapter 13 section II, attempted consolidation and clarification of a tangled mass of law affecting the lives of children. This revision of the law should be considered by child and adolescent psychiatrists in conjunction with prospective revisions of the law concerning divorce, adoption and violence within the family. The guidance and regulations to the Act will be required reading for those providing in-patient psychiatric services for children in secure accommodation and should be considered in relation to the Mental Health Act 1983, England and Wales.

However, the best available practice of child and adolescent psychiatry can continue and be improved irrespective of the legal framework. The Royal College of Psychiatrists has members working in Scotland, the province of Northern Ireland and in Eire, and this book is directed to all within the speciality. Principles for practice remain unchanged and those working in complementary legal systems will wish to apply them as is appropriate. A glossary, by Richard White, on the law in England and Wales, and a selected bibliography are appended.

Acknowledgements

We thank Lady Justice Butler-Sloss for her foreword to the first edition. We are most grateful to Richard White who, besides making specific contributions, read and criticised the manuscript. We thank the assessors of the Royal College of Psychiatrists.

We are most appreciative of the hard work and patience of Diana Hendriks who prepared and sub-edited this revised edition, of Laura Scott, who typed and corrected many drafts of earlier editions, and of Lucretia King for her work as editor.

1 Clinical and forensic child and adolescent psychiatry: forensic second options

This chapter first describes the training and role of child and adolescent psychiatrists and in what areas they may claim to be expert witnesses. It then examines the different ways in which child and adolescent psychiatrists become involved in legal cases, and finally touches upon the ethical issues which must be considered by doctors doing medico-legal work.

The child and adolescent psychiatrist

Child and adolescent psychiatrists are medically trained. This basic training provides them with a grounding in scientific method and its application to research, assessment, observation and treatment in physical and mental disorders. Knowledge of the human body and its anatomy, physiology and pathology lays the foundation for an understanding of the wide range of links between physical and mental disorders. Following qualification there will be a minimum period of one year of work in various medical specialities. Of particular relevance will be the experience of having to cope with emergencies and of dealing with the practical and emotional problems posed by serious illness, disability and death.

After this pre- and post-registration experience the future child and adolescent psychiatrist will enter a formal training scheme in general psychiatry. Many will have preceded this by experience in medicine or paediatrics. The psychiatric training, which leads to the examination for the membership of the Royal College of Psychiatrists, lasts for at least two and a half years; the bulk of this time will be spent working with adult psychiatric patients. The child

1

and adolescent psychiatrist is thus fully qualified to assess the mental state of adult members of any referred family and will know if a member of a family has a disorder which requires and which might be susceptible to treatment.

A doctor who becomes a member of the Royal College of Psychiatrists may apply for a post as specialist registrar in child and adolescent psychiatry. If successful he or she starts on a further training course. The bulk of the trainee's time is devoted to clinical work under supervision. Although specialist registrars may have a special interest in one form of treatment, such as family therapy or individual work with children, they are expected to gain experience in all the different modes of treatment. They will be expected to work in a wide variety of settings including in-patient units, child psychiatric clinics and as a consultant to social service and educational facilities. They will be required to attend a series of seminars and lectures in child development and theoretical aspects of the speciality and to carry out a research project under supervision. On completion of training in an approved scheme the candidate is eligible to apply for a consultant post. In terms of expertise gained, although this will cover child development and family dynamics among other aspects, the basic skill is in the diagnosis and treatment of psychiatric disorders of children. The formal framework for the differential diagnosis and classification of these disorders is set out in internationally recognised systems, ICD–10 (World Health Organization, 1992) and DSM–IV (American Psychiatric Association, 1994). Of particular relevance to legal work is the understanding of the way in which family and other environmental influences can precipitate, worsen or ameliorate these different disorders and their prognosis.

Local and external psychiatric opinions

The majority of child and adolescent psychiatrists work within one trust and will have the responsibility of providing a clinical service for children and families within their catchment area. In the course of this work they will at times be asked to provide a psychiatric report for a court. This may arise in a number of ways. Sometimes the child is known to the psychiatrist before litigation arises. Thus a child already receiving a psychiatric service might subsequently become the subject of a residence or contact dispute between separated parents or the child might commit an offence. A psychiatrist asked under such circumstances to become involved as a *professional witness* in a legal dispute should do so only with the written agreement of both parents, where relevant the child, preferably via joint written instructions and if in doubt should consult a defence society. Written instructions are part of the court documentation and should be made available to all parties.

Other requests will be made for assessment of children unknown to the psychiatrist and his or her colleagues. Most child and adolescent psychiatrists work closely with their local social service departments, offering consultation for its staff and seeing children referred directly by social workers. A request may come from the department asking for an appointment for a child where treatment is not requested but solely an opinion as to whether the child's emotional health will be best met by social services taking a particular action, such as applying for a care order. Similar requests may come from local solicitors, court welfare officers or guardians ad litem. Here one is acting as a professional witness.

This form of involvement can be contrasted with that provided by an 'outside' psychiatrist, one not working in the service local to the child. There are two main reasons for asking such a psychiatrist to provide a court report. First, he or she may be regarded as having special expertise, for example, through having done relevant research. Second, the person requesting the report specifically may wish to obtain an external overview from someone who has no formal links with any of the local services. Sometimes both considerations apply.

Thus, a guardian ad litem may be concerned about the views of the social service department regarding a particular child and about the psychiatric advice given. A parent may disagree with an opinion expressed by a local psychiatrist, for example that a child should not be returned home, and may seek a second opinion. Here one is acting as an expert witness.

On being asked to provide a court report, child and adolescent psychiatrists, whether local or external, should consider whether to agree to become involved and, if so, how. There are many advantages in local psychiatrists undertaking this task. They will know the variety of services and will be in a better position to evaluate the reliability of reports provided. They will know what treatment facilities are available and what it may be realistic to recommend for the child. The clinical assessment may be offered as part of their contractual responsibilities. Such an assessment can be spread over a period of time and can include a trial of treatment. The external consultant may be paid for each item of work conducted, either by one of the parties directly, or through the legal aid system. There may be some pressure for a firm view to be provided after a single interview.

There are, however, disadvantages for a local psychiatrist who rightly may see his or her chief role as providing treatment and consider that a court appearance and the presentation of views unacceptable to parents may jeopardise the chances of continuing treatment. The psychiatrist may be very unhappy about the way social services are conducting a particular case but wish to deal with any disagreement informally or in a case review. If, however, such a psychiatrist were to write a formal report criticising the local social services department this could damage the chances of future collaboration and liaison with the workers involved. In such cases it could be wise to recommend that an outside psychiatrist be approached to provide an assessment for the purposes of a court hearing. To refuse to take part in *any* legal work would however suggest that a full psychiatric service was not being provided for the children in a particular health authority's area.

The provision of psychiatric opinions to local courts is today an essential part of the work of any child and adolescent psychiatrist. However, the provision of court reports and expert evidence per se does not necessarily fall within the contractual obligations of a National Health Service psychiatrist. Clinical assessments undertaken specifically for courts also fall outside contractual duties. Such work must be funded, commissioned and costed separately from contractual work and paid accordingly by those who commissioned it (see Chapter 14).

Independent psychiatrists have a major responsibility not to make therapeutic work more difficult for colleagues in local services. It is a matter of basic courtesy to inform any local psychiatrist who is involved clinically with the child and family that an approach for a second opinion has been made.

It is necessary to consider whether it will be in the child's best interests to have a further diagnostic interview. Repeated assessments can be distressing. They may suggest to a child that he or she is not believed and place that child under great stress. It may be appropriate to suggest that, rather than further interviewing the child, an opinion be given on reports produced locally and possibly on interviews that have been recorded on videotape. If, however, on the basis of information provided, there is potential for differing expert opinions or if initial expert assessment indicates that a child will cope better within a more flexible framework than can be achieved in a single session, there may be no alternative to further interviews. Any form of expert opinion, and the work done in order to formulate it, may be subjected to critical evaluation by cross examination and the writer must be prepared for this process.

Disagreements

The adversarial nature of the court system may lead a psychiatrist, unwisely, to become partisan. Other psychiatrists involved may be seen as being 'on the other side' and consequently wrong. In practice disagreements are usually matters of emphasis, such as on the value of incomplete evidence as to which of two not very satisfactory courses will be better for the child. It is important that one does not attack the integrity of colleagues, but, if there is a disagreement, the reasons for this should be carefully explained. The advantages and disadvantages of one's colleagues' suggestions should be spelt out. The very different roles expected of the local and outside psychiatrist should be detailed and an account given of the effect of these roles on the opinions given. Here the duty to consult colleagues is most helpful.

Ethical issues

Patients or the parents of a patient normally go to a doctor with the understanding that all information given is totally confidential and will be used to help them deal with a particular illness or problem. If, however, an assessment is being undertaken at the request of a third party this duty of confidentiality no longer applies. Any reports being produced become the property of the third party requesting the assessment. It therefore must be explained very carefully to a family what is the nature of the assessment and what will be done with the information received. If, during the course of treatment, the doctor feels that a child is at risk, it would be unethical not to refer to child protection services. Except in the most extreme circumstances here too the parents must be carefully told this is being done and why. An excellent guide to the ethical issues is provided by the General Medical Council (1995) and recent guidelines on the writing of expert reports are given in the next chapter.

Resources

Departments of child and adolescent psychiatry are understaffed in relation to the increasing workload requested of them. Child and adolescent psychiatrists with forensic skills may be helpful in identifying and auditing such service needs and in providing consultation to colleagues. Ideally, with better national manpower levels, they will gain experience in action both as local and external experts and many will develop special interests in particular types of legal work.

International aspects

All countries should attempt to provide for the legal rights, care and welfare of children. The resource implications worldwide are huge.

Children are usually caught up in war and civil conflict, including guerrilla warfare, and acts of terrorism. They may be subjected to persecution, torture and 'disappearances' of family members and of themselves. They may be caught up in man-made and natural disasters such as flood, fire and earthquakes. They and their families and communities may be subjected to famine, and this may be linked with any of the causes listed above. Survivors' health may be damaged by malnutrition or under-nutrition of themselves and their caretakers. Children may suffer negative discrimination on account of their race, skin colour or creed. This may be institutionalised discrimination, where the law requires or empowers it, as has happened in South Africa, Nazi Germany and to many Jewish communities, or may occur where it is neither legally required nor enforced but continues despite the constraint of law. Negative discrimination affecting children may include inadequate provision of housing, schooling, health services or job opportunities and this may occur in any society and between any combination of religious, racial or politically identified groups. For example, migrant workers may be the disadvantaged members of any society which, having imported the workers and their families, itself faces economic pressure.

Children may be dislocated as immigrants, refugees or 'economic refugees' such as the Vietnamese boat children. They may be displaced by man-made or natural disasters or may be offered what are seen as positive economic advantages by adoption from a less wealthy to a more wealthy country. Children may suffer specifically from economic hardship when their work is required for the survival of the family unit. They may be subjected to life-threatening or unhealthy working conditions and offered little or no schooling. Additionally they may be disadvantaged by exposure to malnutrition, infection and pollution. They may be bought or sold for economic or sexual use.

In many societies, children may be subject to repressive legal systems which take no account of their age and status. For example, they may be imprisoned with adults and subjected to harsh and inappropriate punishments, or recruited as soldiers.

Child and adolescent psychiatrists can strive, when training legal and mental health specialists, to provide an international perspective to this training and to consider the civil and legal rights of children locally, nationally and internationally. (See Black *et al* (1997) for an overview of the effect upon children of psychological trauma; see also *The Convention on the Rights of the Child*, General Assembly of the United Nations, 1989.)

Check-list

(a) Local psychiatrists should consider recommending an external forensic expert if:
  (i) it is a complex or rare problem outside their competence
  (ii) their therapeutic relationship with the family may be jeopardised if they have to state an opinion in court
  (iii) their long-term relationship with other agencies may be damaged
  (iv) their relationship with the family has already broken down, or the family has split up, or they may be perceived, with or without reason, as acting partially
  (v) the NHS service would be jeopardised unreasonably by the time that would be taken by the case.
(b) Psychiatrists asked to provide a forensic report should:
  (i) check that they have appropriate permission including that of the relevant court
  (ii) find out whether other court reports are in existence or in preparation
  (iii) consult colleagues who have undertaken the clinical work
  (iv) consider consultation with colleagues who are expert in forensic work
  (v) consider whether they are being asked for an expert opinion on work already undertaken by themselves or others, or to make a further assessment requiring interviews with the child and family
  (vi) understand that, by direction of the High Court, reports must be made available to all parties in civil cases concerning the welfare of children, irrespective of the conclusions and recommendations made
  (vii) make sure that the instructing solicitor, where appropriate, has the authority of the Legal Aid Board to give instructions.
(c) If the referral is accepted, follow the check-list at the end of Chapter 2 (p. 13).

2 Referral and assessment when an expert opinion is requested

The referral

Source of the request

The child and adolescent psychiatrist may be approached for an expert opinion by any of the parties involved in a legal dispute involving children. These may include the local authority, the parents via their solicitor(s), the guardian ad litem, or others such as grandparents who may wish to be represented in the case. Under the terms of the Children Act 1989, permission for any assessment to be used in legal proceedings that involves direct interviewing of the child must be obtained directly from the relevant court. Normally the request for assessment will come after a court Directions Hearing. Letters of instruction may be agreed by all parties and are part of the court record. Reports will be made available to all parties in civil cases other than those involving compensation claims (see Chapter 10). Thus the danger that a report will be quietly filed and possibly a further opinion sought has been greatly lessened. It had in the past even been known for solicitors to attempt to refuse to pay for a report that did not support their case, although this behaviour has been ruled by the High Court to be totally unacceptable (Noble, 1983). More commonly, attempts have been made to find another view which would support the case. This might have been requested from another child and adolescent psychiatrist, an individual from a related profession, such as clinical psychology, or an independent social worker. This manoeuvre not only made a mockery of using psychiatrists but could also be damaging to the child if it involved repeated interviews. Such practice is undesirable.

This change emphasises that, irrespective of who has originally requested the report, child and adolescent psychiatrists should act as independent witnesses with only one aim: to produce a report which in their view will further the interests of the child. Often social workers will have to be reassured that, even though the request for the report came originally from the parents' solicitors, the psychiatrist is not acting for them and will need to hear the views of both parents and social workers if a helpful report is to be produced.

Fees should be negotiated with the referrer at the time of accepting the referral (see Chapter 14). It should always be assumed that a court appearance will be necessary. The dates of the hearing should be established and the case not accepted if attendance will not be possible or if dates cannot be negotiated. It must be confirmed that the assessment can be completed within the timetable established by the court.

Consent of the court

If a child is to be seen it is essential to determine the status of the child and who has parental responsibility. It is good practice to inform all parties about the reasons for requesting an expert opinion. For legal proceedings, it is essential as indicated above to have written confirmation that the agreement of the court has been given for the referral. The report may otherwise be inadmissible and one may not obtain payment.

Conflicts of interest

An opinion may be requested about, for example, contact or residence for a child who had been previously referred with both parents but where, subsequently, the parents have separated. No report should be produced describing the work done unless both parents have stated their agreement in writing. This applies even if the earlier clinical work gave a clear indication of what would be best for the child. In such a case, it should be suggested that only a subpoena or witness summons would enable evidence to be given. If this course is followed, the psychiatrist is free to give an opinion but the evidence should be confined to those matters directly canvassed. The guidelines laid down by the General Medical Council (1995) may be of help here (see Chapter 5). These situations can be extremely difficult, with psychiatrists being torn between the desire to further the best interests of the child and the need to protect information given by a patient or parent in confidence. If there is any doubt about the correct response which should be given, a medical defence society should be consulted.

Necessary information

Referrers may not know how much or how little information they should send the psychiatrist. If they are unclear and ask for help, the following may be sent to them as a guide.

The referral letter should be specific and cover the following areas.

(a) Reason for requesting psychiatric assessment.
(b) Current situation of child/children (including legal status).
(c) How it arose.
(d) Why it arose.
(e) What is the past and present involvement of social service departments and other agencies? What important decisions have been made at case conference or by courts or others? How have the family used any help offered to them?
(f) What plans are social services (if involved) considering?
(g) What is the relevant past history of the child and family?
(h) Enclosure of copies of reports thought to be relevant or helpful, including all medical and psychiatric reports and school reports.

For very young children

(a) Account of developmental progress before and after placement (e.g. motor skills, locomotion, speech, comprehension, social awareness, self-help skills, continence, etc.).
(b) All available recordings of height and weight and growth velocity tables if available (see Hindmarsh & Brook, 1986).

(A report from the health visitor may also help in assessing these and other factors.)

For all children

(a) Description of known behavioural or emotional problems.
(b) Quality of relationships (parents, siblings, adults including other professionals, peers).
(c) School adjustment where relevant (attendance, attainment, ability and behaviour), before and after placement(s).
(d) List of all placements, with dates and details.

Questions to be answered

Referrers should be asked to specify questions they wish answered. The more specific the question, the more likely it is the psychiatrist will be able to help. Examples may be:

(a) Should parental contact continue and, if so, how should this be planned (duration, frequency and place of visits)? If not,

would specific work need to be done with the child to help with relinquishing ties?
(b) Would it be damaging to separate a child from any siblings? Are there advantages in considering separation?
(c) Has the child's emotional development been avoidably impaired, and does he or she require treatment because of this?
(d) Is it likely that sexual abuse has occurred?

In addition, referrers should be encouraged to ask whether significant harm has occurred or may follow any particular action.

Sometimes referral letters can be very vague, asking only for an opinion. It is important to go back to the referrer and ask for a detailed written explanation of what exactly is required in that opinion.

Who should attend for interview?

Careful consideration of this question should take place as soon as the referral is accepted. It is essential to try to see all parties to the dispute. If possible a meeting should be arranged where all, including those professionals involved, can come together and the purpose of the assessment be spelt out (see below). Sometimes this is not possible. The hostility between separated parents may be too great, or a child may not have seen a parent for some time. In these cases a letter should go to all various parties explaining what will be done, who will be seen, and stressing the independence of the assessment. It may happen that pressure is put upon the psychiatrist not to see a particular individual involved in the case. Unless there are acceptable clinical reasons for this, this restriction should not be accepted.

The assessment

The assessment should begin with a brief meeting of all those who have attended for the interview. This may involve the parents, the children, the social worker, foster parents or a lawyer. There should be a discussion about the purpose and nature of the assessment. It must be explained to parents that they and their children are not patients, but that a request has been made for an independent opinion on how the children's needs can be best met, and that a report will be prepared. What will be done throughout the assessment should be described. The independence of the psychiatrist irrespective of who has asked for the assessment and his or her responsibility to the court must be emphasised to all.

In addition to a family interview, the parents and child or children should be seen alone. If in dispute, each parent should be seen independently. A full history should be taken. The parents' views on the case and on their relationship with social workers and others should be obtained. If there is denial that certain incidents have occurred, the parents should be asked to give their accounts. If there are disputes over where a child should live, that child should be seen with all parties, unless there are compelling reasons why this should not take place. Reports, when written, will be made available to all parties who will be entitled to require the expert to attend court for cross-examination.

Techniques of assessment

The basis of any assessment must be a comprehensive evaluation based upon good child psychiatric practice. For the child, the interview may be the first time that they have had the opportunity or have felt safe enough to talk about, or reveal in their play, painful matters. It is important that they leave feeling better than when they entered the consulting room. For many parents this may be the first opportunity they have had to explain in detail their view of the matters under consideration. They should at the very least feel that they have had an open-minded, sympathetic hearing. If at the time of seeing the parents the psychiatrist knows what his or her final conclusion will be, it is good practice to tell the parents this, and explain the reasons for it. In some cases this will produce intense anger and hostility, but in many others they will accept that, even if they do not agree with the point of view put forward, it is being offered with the best interests of their child at heart.

In certain circumstances a specialised individual method of assessment may be thought necessary. In other cases the ability of the family to respond to certain family therapy techniques may be considered as a useful tool. Such techniques should be additional to, and in no way a substitute for, routine evaluation. If the specialised techniques used are ones whose validity has not been fully evaluated, the practitioner should be aware of this, and be prepared to justify their use in court (and thus to those who have been interviewed and their legal representatives).

Marrying findings to the scientific literature

The major part of the assessment and preparation of a report relies on the clinical experience of the psychiatrist. The information gained from the assessment will be evaluated against a general background of clinical work carried out in a variety of settings. In addition, however, it is essential that the findings also be interpreted in the light of the large and ever-growing scientific literature. Many lawyers are now familiar with the main issues debated within the field of developmental psychopathology. Psychiatrists must expect to be questioned on how their opinions fit in with, for example, the literature on attachment or maternal deprivation.

This is clearly not the place to provide a full syllabus of the areas of knowledge that are essential for the expert witness. An introduction to the area, with references for further reading, is provided by Wolkind (1994). There is a need for the practitioner to have a detailed knowledge of the clinical literature. A consultant psychiatrist will normally have received a full training and should be familiar with the contents of the reading list of the Royal College of Psychiatrists. Thus, if the significance of a particular symptom or finding is in question, it should be possible to speak knowledgeably about its prevalence, treatment and prognosis. Should an unusual situation arise, such as whether a child could be better cared for by a mother who has a lesbian relationship or by a father living alone, the relevant research publications should be consulted and presented to the court. If the opinion given in this particular case goes against the findings from research, this must be explained.

Although much of what child and adolescent psychiatrists practise necessarily must have an intuitive and subjective element, it is essential to emphasise the large scientific basis to the speciality and to use this to offer guidance to courts on the alternatives facing a child. The evidence of psychiatrists may be important in helping courts establish the definitions of significant harm and responsible parenting.

Check-list

This list is for use when speaking or writing to referrers.

(a) Understand who is requesting your opinion and on whose behalf.
(b) Ascertain who is the legal guardian of the child(ren).
(c) Make sure there is no conflict of interest for you in agreeing to the request to give an opinion.
(d) Ensure you have the permission of the court to see the child(ren).
(e) Request (and make sure you receive) necessary reports and information.
(f) Clarify what questions you are being asked.
(g) Clarify whom you wish to interview.
(h) Allow enough time for interviews and writing the report.
(i) Consider the relevant scientific literature.
(j) Check that you are available at the time of the court hearing.
(k) Negotiate fees.

3 Reporting for the court

Writing a clear and helpful report is the most important and difficult part of a psychiatric assessment. The lawyer's view of a witness will be determined by the way facts and arguments are presented. The contents of a report will provide the basis for an examination in court. A thoughtful and convincing report may lead to the withdrawal of the case, or to an attempt to arrange a compromise between the parties rather than a full hearing.

The report should be as brief as is compatible with the complexity of the case. It should be typed, double spaced on headed paper with large margins, and dated and signed. It should be concise, readable and devoid of jargon. This latter point is particularly important. In clinical work, terms are often used which have never been validated by formal research, but which represent subjective impression and can be helpful shorthand devices for discussions with colleagues. Examples would be 'enmeshment' or 'network' or 'poor ego strength'. This is psychiatric jargon and should be avoided in reports. Other words can be seen as technical. If taken for granted and undefined, they too will become jargon. Thus if the term 'insecure attachment' is used, its meaning should be explained, the observations made should be described and an opinion given as to their significance.

Before final typing, the report should be re-read to eliminate jargon which has been overlooked. Examples of reports varying in style are given in the second part of the book. None is perfect, but all would be helpful to those who have to make decisions about a child. This chapter gives various headings which, if used, would conduct the reader of the report through the assessment and demonstrate how the writer came to the conclusions.

Principles for practice

Mr (now Lord) Justice Thorpe (1993) provided the following principles for practice, based on recent judgements:

(a) Medical experts must be impartial, involved with the leave of the court, independent and accurate.

(b) Key adults in the child's life should not be identified when this is not in the interests of the child (an important principle given that reports as indicated above are now distributed to all parties in a case. This procedure should not identify inappropriately information private to the child and his representatives).

(c) In family proceedings the expert's sole concern must be the welfare of the child. In an important recent decision he made clear that in children's cases professional privilege did not extend to experts' reports (*Essex County Council* v. *R* [1993] 2 FLR 826), emphasising the statement also made by Mr Justice Wall (Tufnell, 1995) that in children's cases reports must be made available to all parties.

(d) Interviews should be limited in number. There are dangers of muddling investigation and therapy. Recommendations made in the Cleveland Report (Butler-Sloss, 1988) should be considered carefully.

(e) The principle now contained in a recent Court of Appeal decision (Re *M and R* [1996] 2 FLR 195) is as follows: "Expert evidence on whether a child is telling the truth is admissible, but the relevance of that evidence, and the weight to be attached to it, as with the ultimate decision, are matters for the judge".

(f) The obligation of an expert is to stick to a brief given by the court and not, without further discussion and agreement, to go beyond the parameters agreed in instructions.

(g) The Children (Admissibility of Hearsay Evidence) Order 1993 provides that hearsay evidence shall be admissible, in all three tiers of court, in relation to the upbringing of a child.

Assessment

The court has jurisdiction to order or prohibit any assessment that involves the participation of the child. This power is directed to providing the court with the material that, in the view of the court, was required to enable it to reach a proper decision at the final hearing of the application for a care order. The House of Lords has held that although the relevant Children Act guidance refers to the examination or assessment of the child, a child could not be divorced from its environment, so that a court can make a direction, requiring the assessment of a child, which also includes another relevant person. The court could dictate the placement of the child during an interim care order for the purposes of an assessment and could direct the authority to fund any necessary placement, although it would take into account the cost and the fact that the local authority resources were limited. The court may not order that a child live with his or her parents during the course of an interim care order, which is a discretion vested in the local authority (see Re *C (Interim Care Order: Residential Assessment)* [1997] 1 FLR 1).

Instruction and preparation of expert witnesses

Mr Justice Wall in a recent judgement provided guidance (Tufnell, 1995) endorsed and amplified by the Children Act Advisory Committee (1994–1995) and summarised as follows:

(a) It is essential that medical experts asked to give reports or opinions on child care cases are fully instructed with appropriate permission of the court. The letter of instruction should always set out the context in which the expert's opinion is sought and define carefully the specific questions the expert has been asked to address. Joint instruction by all parties is recommended.

(b) Careful thought should be given to the selection of the papers sent to the expert with the letter of instruction, which always should list the documents which are being sent. "A doctor who ventures an opinion on inadequate material is taking a substantial risk that his or her opinion may be unsound."

(c) Where an expert's report is put in evidence the letter of instruction to the expert should always be disclosed to the other parties and included in the bundle of documents to be used in court. Experts should expect to receive each other's reports.

(d) Doctors and other experts should not hesitate to request further information and ask for additional documentation. An expert should make clear the limits of his expertise.

(e) Doctors who have had clinical experience of the child or children outside the immediate remit of the litigation (for example a paediatrician who has examined or treated a child prior to the proceedings being taken) should carefully review their notes before writing a court report and ensure that all the clinical material is available for inspection by the court and by other experts called upon to advise in the case. This includes (although this is not an exhaustive list) all medical notes, hospital records, photographs, correspondence and X-rays.

(f) Experts who are going to be called to give evidence at the trial must keep up-to-date with developments in the case relevant to their opinion (and it is the duty of the instructing solicitor or solicitors to facilitate this). "There is nothing more embarrassing for an expert (as well as time-wasting in court) than to be confronted with a document or piece of evidence with which he or she has not previously been supplied, which he or she needs time to consider and which may vitiate the opinion previously expressed in writing" (Mr Justice Wall quoted in Tufnell, 1995). If an opinion nevertheless is based on insufficient data, or is changed in the light of new evidence, this must be made explicit. Opinions based on research must be identified as such.

(g) Experts should always be invited to confer with each other, by the guardian ad litem if available, or else by the instructing solicitors, pre-trial in an attempt to reach agreement where possible and to identify remaining areas in contention. It is preferable that this discussion should be reported to the court in written form.

(h) Careful cooperative planning between the legal advisers to the different parties in an early stage of the preparation for the trial should be undertaken to ensure the experts' availability and that they can be called to give evidence in a logical sequence.

(h) Where an expert's opinion is uncontentious and she or he is not required for cross-examination, that fact should be established as early as possible in the course of preparation for trial and the expert notified.

Writing the report

A questionnaire survey of good practice in the preparation of expert witness reports was undertaken by Tufnell & Cottrell (1995), with guidance from other sources including advice from the British Juvenile and Family Courts Association and support and cooperation from the Lord Chancellor's Department, the Official Solicitor to the Supreme Court, the National Association of Guardians ad Litem and the Association of Lawyers for Children. (See also Tufnell, 1993; Tufnell & Cottrell, 1996.)

The results of this questionnaire study have resulted in a recommended format of experts' reports prepared by Peter Harris, Official Solicitor, and reproduced in full as follows. Although it specifically refers to reports for the Official Solicitor, the format can usefully be applied to other reports for court.

Experts' reports: format in children cases

This note is for the guidance of expert witnesses who are instructed by the Official Solicitor, and has been based upon the research undertaken by Tufnell and Cottrell (Tufnell & Cottrell, 1995, 1996; Cottrell & Tufnell, 1996). It is essentially a matter for each expert to decide how best to present his or her report to the Official Solicitor in a way which will be most helpful to him and to the court, in the light of the Official Solicitor's instructions and in the context of the proceedings. However, the following suggestions regarding the format of a report are likely to assist in achieving that end, and in providing a report which lends itself to being rapidly assimilated.

Summary of preferred report layout

Large typeface.
Double spacing.
A4 sheets, page numbered.
Short sentences; short paragraphs.
Numbered paragraphs and sections.
Headed sections.
Clear English, avoiding technical terms.
Separate sections for summary, conclusions and recommendations.
Less than 20 pages.
Table of contents if more than eight pages.
Details of interviews, documents seen, etc. in appendices.

Structure and content

The first page of the report should include the:

Nature of proceedings and court reference number.
Title of the document and date made.
Subject's name, date of birth, age when interviewed and status (e.g. applicant, respondent, child subject).
Author's name, qualifications, position and area of expertise.
Author's address, telephone number, etc.

(It is helpful for this page also to be used, in reverse, as backing for the report, since this facilitates identification in court proceedings.)

This should be followed by an introductory section covering the following:

> Relevant amplifying information about the author.
> Identify report as one written for the Official Solicitor, giving synopsis of reasons for making the report (or in other contexts identify reasons for writing the report).
> Refer to the letter(s) of instruction.
> Synopsis of sources of information, giving a full list of these in an appendix.

Then set out relevant background information, for example:

> A summary of the facts.
> Identify the sources of information.
> Set out hypotheses guiding the assessment.

Following the background give an account of your assessment, including:

> Interviews, factual information about the child, parents, other carers, family, etc.
> Facts obtained through other investigations.
> Summarise main findings of your assessment.

> (It is most important that your report states clearly the facts upon which your assessment is based and the inferences which you feel able to draw from those facts.)

Next give your opinion, dealing with the following, as appropriate:

> Your general diagnostic conclusions about the child and family.
> A psychiatric/psychological diagnosis of the child.
> Identification of resources necessary to meet the child's needs.
> Comment on what legal orders might be beneficial to the child.
> Answers to questions posed in letter(s) of instruction.

Finally, end the report with your recommendations. In a report of any substance it will be desirable briefly to explain the options which you believe may be considered. You should deal with the pros and cons of each, or any, option which you have invited the court to consider. However, it is usually important to provide one unequivocal set of recommendations.

The report must be signed and dated, below a statement (required by Rules of Court) which reads:

I declare that this statement is true to the best of my knowledge, information and belief, and I understand that it may be placed before the Court.

Conclusion

Mr (now Lord) Justice Thorpe (1994) summarised the aims of partnership between child and adolescent psychiatrists and court as follows:

The decisions to be made by judges could be incredibly taxing but that burden was lightened by sharing it with expert witnesses. The expert would have penetrated the home family scene, something to which the judge was never exposed directly. That was in one sense a safeguard; but a price was paid in not reaching the heart of family life, a deficiency made good by the experts' input.

Check-list

(a) Use headed paper and date it.
(b) Include an opening.
(c) Include an introduction.
(d) Include a history from reports.
(e) Include a history from informants.
(f) Include an account of your assessment.
(g) Include other investigations.
(h) Include a summary.
(i) Include your opinion.
(j) Include recommendations.
(k) Sign the report, and include your qualifications and professional positions.
(l) Append or include lists of documents read, appointments offered, inquiries made, and other relevant reports.

Note that the Children Act 1989 has now provided courts with a check-list (see p. 106). Your report should address itself to these points, using them as headings where appropriate.

(a) Ascertainable wishes of the child.
(b) Physical, emotional and educational needs.
(c) The likely effect on the child of any change in his/her circumstances.
(d) Age, gender, background, etc.
(e) Harm suffered or at risk of being suffered.

(f) Capability of adults concerned of meeting child's needs.
(g) Powers of the court.

Significant case references

1. Re *G (Children's cases: Instruction of Experts)* [1994] 2 FLR 291.
2. Re *M (Minors) (Care Proceedings: Child's Wishes)* [1994] 1 FLR 749 (requirement of experts to discuss reports prior to a hearing).
3. *Oxfordshire County Council* v. *M* [1994] 1 FLR 175.
4. Re *MD and TD (Minors) (Time Estimates)* [1994] 2 FLR 336 (need for effective timetabling).
5. *Essex County Council* v. *R* [1993] 2 FLR 826 (professional privilege not extended to experts' reports in child cases).
6. *X (Minors)* v. *Bedfordshire County Council*; *M (A Minor) and Another* v. *Newham London Borough Council and Others*; *E (A Minor)* v. *Dorset County Council*; *Christmas* v. *Hampshire County Council*; *Keating* v. *Bromley London Borough Council* [1995] 2 FLR 276. Appeals in two child abuse and three education cases were heard together.

   The common theme was a claim on behalf of the children based on breach of statutory duty or common law negligence by a local authority. Either: a local authority had failed properly to investigate allegations of abuse or it had failed to provide appropriate services.

   The appeals relating to breach of statutory duty were dismissed and no common law duty was owed in respect of negligence.

   In the education cases (Dorset, Hampshire and Bromley) local authorities owed no direct common law duty of care in the exercise of powers and discretions relating to children with special needs conferred by the Education Acts 1944–1981.

   However, authorities could be liable in relation to the operation and provision of educational services.
7. In Re *C (Detention: Medical Treatment)* [1997] 2 FLR 180 Mr Justice Wall held that a child suffering from anorexia nervosa may be required by order under the inherent jurisdiction of the High Court to undergo relevant therapeutic treatment while resident in a designated clinic.
8. The House of Lords has recently considered whether a child who suffers harm following alleged negligence by a local authority has a remedy in damages at [1995] 3 All ER 353. In *M* v. *London Borough of Newham*, the parents alleged that child had been taken into care after an inadequate investigation into allegations of harm. In *X* v. *Bedfordshire County Council*, the

position was reversed. The authority did not take care proceedings and the child was subsequently harmed.

The House of Lords held that a child had no cause of action for harm arising from: (a) an alleged failure of a local authority to comply with its statutory duties under children's welfare legislation; (b) careless performance of a statutory duty has no cause of action against the authority nor would any action lie in negligence in respect of an alleged failure; (c) actions or decisions where a common law duty of care might arise, if they came within the ambit of a statutory discretion. If they were so unreasonable as to fall outside the ambit, there could be a common law liability. The authority might be liable for negligent misstatement, even though it could not be liable for breach of statutory duty. In May 1998 the European Commission of Human Rights declared that both *X* v. *Bedfordshire County Council* and *M* v. *London Borough of Newham* were admissible applications. The Commission will now consider the merits of the applications and place itself at the disposal of the parties with a view to securing a friendly settlement. If a solution is not reached, the Commission will state its opinion as to whether the facts disclose a breach by the Government of their obligations under the European Convention of Human Rights (article 31). The Report will be transmitted to the Committee of Ministers, which will decide the matter unless the case is referred to the European Court of Human rights by the Commission on the UK Government. *T* v. *Surrey County Council* [1994] 2 FCR 1269, a case relating to a registered childminder held to have injured a child in her care. This decision might now be considered under (b) or (c).

Followed in *H* v. *Norfolk County Council* [1997] 1 FLR 384, but distinguished in the Court of Appeal in *Barrett* v. *Enfield LBC* [1997] 2 FLR 167, where duties were said to be owed by a local authority to a child in care.

4 Court procedure

Once involved in preparing a report, a child and adolescent psychiatrist should assume that he or she will be asked to give evidence in court. In some instances, no appearance in person will be required. The principle is that written reports are not, by themselves, admissible as evidence without the witness being available for examination and cross-examination, with two specific exceptions (for medical purposes). These are: (a) the Education Act 1996, section 566 – a certificate issued and signed by a medical officer of a local education authority shall be received in evidence; and (b) the Children and Young Persons Act 1963, section 26 – a written report is admissible if certified by a qualified medical practitioner as to the physical or mental condition of any person. This provision enables any doctor to give details of injuries in writing and possibly to avoid attendance at the interim stage of care proceedings. It is appropriate for doctors in these circumstances to check with the instructing solicitor as to whether they may report in this way. If an opinion is to be expressed, as to the cause of injuries, the doctor is also likely to have to attend. In all courts, evidence is admissible by report and witness statement, but if the judge or magistrates wish to ask any questions on the report or if the evidence is challenged by any of the parties, the psychiatrist will be required to attend and give oral evidence.

Court attendance can be inconvenient and it may lead to the cancellation of hospital clinics or other activities. It is best to agree voluntarily to go to court and negotiate as early as possible for the least difficult time. Courts are normally very helpful, recognising the demands on a doctor's time, and will try, within reason, to cause as little inconvenience as possible. If requests by lawyers for a suitable time are ignored, they may be driven to issue a witness summons or subpoena to compel attendance. Even if this is issued with very little notice, it must be obeyed otherwise one may be held to be in contempt of court. It is far better to avoid this situation.

The evidence given in court will depend on whether the psychiatrist is there as a professional or as an expert witness. In the former an account is required based solely on first-hand knowledge of the dealings the psychiatrist has had with the child and the family. Opinions may of course be given, such as the reasons for the failure of treatment, or how disturbed the child was compared with others seen in similar situations, but basically what is required is an account of the psychiatrist's direct clinical work. Case notes may be brought and referred to, but quotes from them will be admissible only if they were made contemporaneously.

In contrast or in addition the expert witness, who may not have even seen the child (see Chapter 1), will be expected to comment on general issues relevant to the case and to evaluate the views of others involved. In practice the division between the two sorts of witnesses may not be as sharp as implied here. It would not be unreasonable for professional witnesses, if they are experienced consultants, also to be treated as expert witnesses. They may be asked to expand their evidence and to comment on issues outside of their direct involvement in the case. Expert witnesses too should bring their original notes to the court and demonstrate that they can clearly differentiate between pieces of information heard or observed and the interpretation of that information.

Evidence should always be based on a report submitted in advance and seen by all the lawyers, parties and the judge or magistrates. If new evidence comes to light during the case, this can of course be presented but, even here, if possible, a supplementary report should be prepared, to enable all parties to evaluate the significance of the additional factors. Most solicitors are happy for medical reports to be submitted in their original form. Others insist on a sworn affidavit. If this is demanded, this should be a brief statement identifying the report as one's own, and the report should be exhibited to the affidavit. Any attempts to turn the entire report into an affidavit should be resisted. The intended nuances of the psychiatric report can easily be lost in the process of 'translation' into legal language. The statement that the report is believed to be true and known to be available to a court of law must be appended in the form of words outlined in the previous chapter.

Expert witnesses are at times asked to sit in court and listen to the proceedings so that their evidence can include comments on testimony heard during the proceedings. Barristers and solicitors often discuss evidence as it is given, with the psychiatrist sitting in court, acting in the additional role of psychiatric adviser to counsel. Although time-consuming, this could be justified in extremely complex or difficult cases, such as are heard in the High Court. This role may also be expected of the psychiatrist, although less often, in county and family proceedings courts.

The Children Act 1989 aimed at reforming the law dealing with children rather than the court structure but it has made important changes to the jurisdiction and procedures of the courts.

Jurisdiction in all proceedings under the Act is concurrent and cases may be transferred, under rules made by the Lord Chancellor, between tiers of court or between courts in the same tier. The Act also enabled the creation of a magistrates' court for family proceedings, staffed by a family court panel. The aim has been to create a flexible system where cases may be heard according to their complexity and length, to enable all proceedings affecting the same child, or children of the same family where necessary, to be heard in the same court and at the same time, and to make sure that the magistrates and judges who do this work have made a special study of and are experienced in family law.

In January 1995 the President of the Family Division, Sir Stephen Brown, issued a direction on case management which recognised the importance of reducing cost and delay in civil litigation. The court must exercise discretion to limit: (a) discovery; (b) the length of opening and closing oral submissions; (c) the time allowed for the examination and cross-examination of witnesses; (d) the issues on which it wishes to be addressed; and (e) reading aloud from documents and authorities. The President directed that unless otherwise ordered, every witness statement or affidavit shall stand as the evidence in chief of the witness concerned.

> The substance of the evidence which a party intends to adduce at the hearing must be sufficiently detailed, but without prolixity; it must be confined to material matters of fact, not, (except in the case of the evidence of professional witnesses) of opinion; and if hearsay evidence is to be adduced, the source of the information must be declared or good reason given for not doing so.

But parties and legal representatives owe a duty to the court to give full and frank disclosure "in all matters in respect of children". Parties and their advisers must use their best endeavours to: (a) confine issues and evidence to what is reasonably considered to be essential; (b) reduce or eliminate issues for expert evidence; and (c) to agree in advance which are the issues or main issues to be considered.

There are directions about the preparation of bundles of evidence, in A4 format where possible and suitably secured. Such bundles must be lodged with a court at least two days before a hearing – paginated, indexed, legible and chronologically arranged.

A pre-trial review is recommended for cases estimated to last for five days or more and a chronology and brief 'skeleton argument' summarising the submissions of each party and citing main authorities to be relied upon, should be lodged with the court. This guidance is issued with the concurrence of the Lord Chancellor and it is in this context that each expert witness must consider and present evidence.

Presenting oneself in court

It is vital to arrive in court in good time, although, once there, long delays can often be expected. It is useful to bring some work that could be done should there be delay. In practice the level of tension outside the courts is such that a novel or crossword puzzle would actually be more realistic! Some time should be set aside to meet with solicitors, barristers and other relevant parties before the court hearing. A great deal of legal bargaining takes place just before the court proceedings begin and an agreed course of action satisfying all or some of those in dispute can save time and help the court focus on the more important issues. Expert witnesses may be invaluable in such negotiations. It is usually possible for the child and adolescent psychiatrist's evidence to be heard within an agreed half-day.

Dress and demeanour are important. Courts expect sober, traditional clothes which befit members of a learned profession. It is important for the witness to stand erect, speak distinctly, sufficiently loudly, and with authority. Speak slowly, as the judge may be making notes. If this is the case, it is helpful to watch the speed of the pen or use of a word processor.

The oath is taken, as customary, according to the religious views of the witness, who may, if a non-believer, prefer to affirm. The taking of the oath should be treated very seriously and the witness should look towards the judge or magistrates. The same form should be used in court and when swearing to an affidavit.

High Court judges should be addressed as 'Your Lordship' or 'Your Ladyship' or 'My Lady', or 'My Lord', all other judges as 'Your Honour', and magistrates and district judges as 'Sir' or 'Madam'. When in doubt, consult your instructing solicitor or counsel. The witness will at first be examined (examination-in-chief) by the lawyer acting for those who have sought an opinion. When this is completed lawyers from the other parties will carry out a cross-examination. Following this cross-examination, the first lawyer may ask for a brief re-examination. The judge or magistrates may then ask their own questions. You should face the barrister or solicitor when being asked a question, but should give all your evidence facing the judge or magistrate. If you feel that you are being bullied or harassed, or if you are aware that the matter is irrelevant or delicate, or has been already dealt with, and no objection is lodged by the non-examining counsel or the judge, you can ask for a ruling from the judge, or from the chairman of the magistrates, as to whether the question is relevant or necessary to answer. You may wish to argue that some information may be hurtful to people in court, or unnecessary to the case. You should be mindful of the feelings of parents (for example) who will usually be present, and use your skill to phrase matters in the least damaging way at all times.

It is important to keep in mind the need to provide a considered opinion based on facts and current medical knowledge. The presence or absence of psychiatric disorder, in child or parent, may be a central issue. It may be appropriate to deal with causative factors which are associated with particular conditions and events which precipitate and maintain disorders. Adequacy of parental care, appropriateness of the child's school, environment, and the influence of environmental factors in the child's life may require comment. The outcome of psychiatric disorder is often a relevant topic, as is the availability and likely response to appropriate treatment.

Sometimes the consequences of possible placements will require discussion, for example a child's possible response to foster care, special schools or a children's home. The court wishes to hear the opinion of an experienced practitioner well used to working with disturbed children. When giving oral evidence, relevant psychiatric literature to support an opinion can be quoted. This should be as succinct as possible. Evidence should always be clear, well-thought-out and understandable to the layman.

Factors affecting the normal development of a child or adolescent are relevant. Satisfactory parenting is also an important part of the remit of a child and adolescent psychiatrist (a useful book has been edited by Reder & Lucey, 1995). In many cases, subjects outside the direct current expertise of the child and adolescent psychiatrist may be of importance. These might include adult mental illness, drug misuse or learning disability. Child and adolescent psychiatrists should inform themselves of the relevant condition and present views on its treatment and prognosis. They should make it clear that they are not specialists in the particular field, but that they are still able to give an opinion. Advice from a colleague in the relevant speciality may be quoted. The issues involved are rarely so important that the case would be advanced by hearing from a succession of doctors, each dealing with a very small part of the evidence. If, however, the relevant issue is clearly vital, for example as to whether a parent really will be made well within three months by a new drug regime, then the child and adolescent psychiatrist must insist to the instructing solicitor that a further expert has to be called.

Information received from colleagues such as social workers, psychotherapists, psychologists, teachers, paediatricians, nurses and others can be used to add to your own observations in forming an opinion and may be quoted and acknowledged as part of the evidence.

The psychiatric witness must arrive in court well prepared. Familiarity with all the affidavits and other reports is important. Information which is not available or not yet available, such as school reports or comments by staff at a family centre, must be kept in mind as an unknown and commented upon as such. In an adversarial legal system such as ours opinions will differ, so that contradictory evidence should come as no surprise. If a new fact is presented, it is important to agree that this could modify your original opinion. It is essential to say so when you do not have the answer to a question. It is far better to admit to ignorance of either a detail of the history, or a point of theoretical importance, than to pretend to greater knowledge than you have. Be prepared for psychiatric texts to be quoted against you by cross-examining counsel. If you are unfamiliar with the work say so and ask for time to read it, ensuring that the passage is not being taken out of context. It may be helpful to anticipate possible lines of cross-examination.

Do not feel you need always accept the language in which counsel expresses a question – it may be that you can rephrase it in a way which will actually be more relevant or appropriate to the issue. Similarly, do not hesitate to ask, through the Bench, for clarification of counsel's questions. Do not be afraid to take your time about considering your answer, referring to notes if necessary.

It is vital not to be persuaded to step outside the boundaries of your professional expertise. It is easy to become caught up in the adversarial atmosphere of the court. You must however remain detached from this and admit the flaws and doubts which might exist in the case being presented by the side on whose behalf you are appearing and, when warranted, acknowledge merit in opposing opinions.

At all times you should be aware of the effects that your testimony could have on the child and family. Unfortunately, it is often necessary to spell out in their presence all the difficulties affecting the individuals subject to proceedings. This may sometimes be avoided if judges obtain agreement between counsel that evidence may be presented in the absence of a particular family member who, it is argued, might be harmed by hearing it. However, being excluded from court is upsetting also, and many parents appreciate their 'day in court', feeling they have had a hearing. Court hearings, well conducted, may be cathartic and therapeutic to parties wearied by long conflict.

Attending court can be a stressful experience. Never treat it lightly. It is not uncommon in complex cases to be in the witness box for many hours or even days, and cross-examination by a skilled barrister, while usually conducted courteously, can be extremely tiring and may be quite disturbing. It is helpful to arrange a 'debriefing' session afterwards, either with the solicitor or with a colleague.

If you give your evidence clearly and confidently but not dogmatically, and if you are always courteous and patient, you have nothing to fear and will have done your best to help the child whose future is being decided.

Check-list

(a) Check the date and time of the hearing and the location of the court.
(b) Ensure you are dressed correctly.
(c) Take the relevant files and re-read them in advance.
(d) Read the relevant psychiatric literature if you have not done so recently.
(e) Prepare yourself to anticipate possible lines of cross-examination.
(f) Clarify in your own mind the boundaries of your expertise.

Afterwards:
(g) Arrange a 'debriefing' with a trusted colleague.
(h) Prepare a fee account to be submitted to your instructing solicitor.

5 Confidentiality and consent

Published guidelines

The General Medical Council (1995) has revised and simplified its former guidelines and *Duties of a Doctor* has been circulated to all medical practitioners.

These guidelines, although essential reading, and of the first importance, do not address in detail the range of clinical, ethical and legal issues relevant to child and adolescent psychiatrists working as members of multi-disciplinary teams, with legal minors and in settings outside of the NHS. The following extract from an article by the Royal College of Psychiatrists (1987) is retained in abbreviated form in this new edition as an overview of principles for good practice which remains relevant.

Current concerns of child and adolescent psychiatric teams

This document, by a sub-group of the Child and Adolescent Psychiatry Specialist Section Executive Committee [of the Royal College of Psychiatrists] discusses:
  (i) The right of an NHS patient to confidentiality.
 (ii) The right of a medically qualified member of a multi-disciplinary team to maintain patient confidentiality.
(iii) The right of a patient to access to information about himself as recorded by medical members of multi-disciplinary teams.

Introduction

Child psychiatric teams may include, in addition to NHS employees, social workers, psychologists and teachers employed by local authorities, and additionally they may work conjointly, on specific cases, with probation officers employed by the Home Office, guardians ad litem, children's solicitors, etc. They may also be asked to provide expert evidence in courts of law.

Besides working in NHS bases such as health centres and hospitals, child and adolescent psychiatrists work in local education authority clinics and may contribute, individually or as members of multi-disciplinary teams, to work in prisons or remand centres, secure units, assessment centres, children's homes and schools. They may be asked to contribute to the work of trust disability teams, teams specialising in child protection, adoption and fostering services and divorce court welfare and conciliation services. Information is sensitive and might be obtained from third parties.

Child clients

The client may be a child under the age of 16 years, a young person over 16 years of age who is a legal minor but able, within the terms of the Family Law Reform Act (England and Wales) 1969 section 8, to give consent to medical treatment as though he had reached the age of full majority, or a parent or guardian of such a child. When a child is in the care of a local authority a social worker may, as its agent, act as guardian so far as consent is concerned. Information may be requested about such clients or consent to treatment may be requested. It is good practice to obtain the consent of a parent or guardian for any medical treatment of a young person under 16 years of age and, according to the child's age and understanding, also to obtain his consent.

Young people over 16 years of age can consent to their own treatment and, as far as possible, consent should also be sought for the active involvement of their parents and guardians. The rights of other members of family groups such as siblings and grandparents, co-habitees, step-parents, divorced non-custodial parents, etc., are less clear and should be a matter of careful evaluation at the time of professional assessment. [There is no right to veto treatment to which 16- or 17-year-olds give consent (White, 1995). Consent to treatment in childhood and adolescence has been reviewed by Pearce (1995).]

Confidentiality may be over-ruled where any child is considered to have been abused or to have been at risk of abuse. Standard child abuse procedures apply under such circumstances and all workers must recognise their responsibility to follow Department of Health and Welsh Office or other relevant guidelines. Chapter 13 discusses psychiatric or other medical examinations within the framework of the Children Act 1989 guidelines on child abuse.

Multi-disciplinary teams: record-keeping

Where there is a component from a health professional to notes made by employees of the local authority, social workers, education psychologists, teachers, etc., permission must be obtained from the relevant health professional before information is released. If this is not forthcoming, the information must be removed from the record before access is permitted. Thus the situation seems clear as far as written notes are concerned. What is more difficult is that, for effective multi-disciplinary team working, confidential information obtained by health professionals must be shared with social workers and educationalists. It is essential that methods be found to ensure that such information is not disseminated without the consent of the health professional and the patient and/or parent or guardian.

Maintenance and storage of records

These may be written case notes, computerised information and video and audio tapes. Managers and practitioners in child and adolescent psychiatric services must consider how the records are stored and maintained, how long they should be kept, bearing in mind the possibility of longitudinal research, who has access to them and with what authority. Medical records may be subpoenaed whether they are written or in the form of video or audio tapes.

Patient access to notes

It is the view of the Royal College of Psychiatrists that a patient's access to his notes (this includes parental access to records of legal minors) should be at the discretion of the doctor concerned and not allowed to the patient as of right. Care must be taken not to reveal confidential information concerning third parties or, in many cases, provided by them. (This principle for good practice is modified by the Access to Health Records Act 1990, discussed on p. 33.)

Prospective practice

A substantial burden falls on individual health authorities and local authorities who are required to establish guidelines on confidentiality. The Department of Health is recommended to be involved only when research is under consideration. Yet it is appropriate, where legal minors are concerned, that trusts and local authorities receive central guidance from the Department of Health and the Department for Education and that these issues be debated by professional bodies as well as by employing authorities.

Guidelines

These are available from the General Medical Council, from a DES/DHSS joint circular 1983 (Department of Health and Social Security, 1983*a*) and from the Korner Committee (1984). The Royal College of Psychiatrists has made available relevant discussion documents and working party reports (Baldwin *et al*, 1976; Royal College of Psychiatrists, 1981, 1990).

The Department of Health issues guidance and regulations on child abuse, non-accidental injury and children in substitute family care which should be available to those working in child mental health services. These are revised from time to time and should be placed in departmental libraries.

Access to health records

Relevant legislation

(a) The Data Protection Act 1984, section 21, allows patients access to health records kept on computer, although some information is exempted by the Data Protection (Subject Access Modification) (Health) Order 1987.

(b) The Access to Personal Files Act 1987 gives individuals access to records not held on computer (manual records) held by local authority and local social services authorities but is relevant specifically only to housing and social services functions. Record-keeping by members of multi-disciplinary teams which include health professionals remains as discussed earlier in this chapter.

(c) The Access to Medical Reports Act 1988 requires that an employer or an insurance company cannot see a medical report on an individual for employment or insurance purposes without the knowledge and consent of the individual about whom the report is written. That individual has a right to see the report before the doctor commissioned to prepare it passes it to the relevant employer or insurance company. The individual has also the right to request that corrections be made and may refuse permission for it to be sent to an employer or insurance company.

(d) The Access to Health Records Act 1990, which resulted from a Private Member's Bill, was effective from 1 November 1991. It gives individuals the prospective right of access, subject to search and exemptions, to information about themselves recorded manually in health records. This right of access is similar to that for computerised records existing under the Data Protection Act 1984, as indicated above. The Act does not change or restrict voluntary arrangements between doctor and patient regarding the sharing of information, and principles to be considered by child mental health professionals remain as indicated in this chapter. Principles for forensic psychiatric practice also are unchanged. Guidelines to the Act and other relevant circulars provided from time to time by the Department of Health should be read by all practitioners. The Act applies to NHS records and equally to those within the private health sector and to employers who hold information relevant to the physical or mental health of their employees.

'Holder' is defined within the Act and may be a general practitioner or family practitioner committee, a health professional or a health service body. The 'patient' in relation to a health record is the individual in connection with whose care the record has been made. 'Health professional', also defined within the Act, covers a range of people who provide health care and who have 'professional qualifications'.

Application for access may be made by the patient, a person authorised in writing to make the application on behalf of the patient, and in England and Wales, the person having parental responsibility for a child (under the age of 16 years), or in Scotland, the parent or guardian of a child with pupil status (under the age of 12 years for girls, 14 years for boys). A court may appoint a person to represent a patient incapable of managing his or her own affairs and, where a patient has died, a personal representative or any person who may have a claim arising out of the patient's death may apply for access to records.

The British Medical Association (1991) has prepared guidelines on the Act and provides advice to individual doctors (see also Richardson & Harris-Hendriks, 1996).

Discussion

The medical profession has long had concerns about the possible effects on patient care of statutory right of patient access to health records and is concerned that arrangements for access must have adequate safeguards for patients, doctors, other health professionals and third parties who have contributed to health records.

Among doctors the preference has been for voluntary arrangements between doctor and patients, and it has been argued that legislation is not the correct way to deal with this important issue. The preference was for a voluntary code of practice that could be carefully monitored and adjusted in the light of experience with the individual needs of patients (British Medical Association, 1991). Clinical experience confirms this view.

Child and adolescent psychiatrists, particularly the majority now involved in forensic work, and all who practise within multi-disciplinary teams, probably are well placed to deal with new legislation since they have thought through the issues involved in relation to current practice. In summary, they should bear in mind the issues discussed earlier in this chapter, the guidance on the preparation of psychiatric reports outlined in Chapter 2, and take particular account, in the guidance and regulations, of the delicate relationship between the health professional, the holder of the records, who may be a non-medically qualified employer within the health service, the rights of the child, the rights of the parent and the rights of third parties, who in family assessment work are of course numerous. All work, as ever, should take place within a framework of the highest standards of ethical practice.

In well-conducted practice, it has become clear that formal application within a legal framework for access to records is a rarity. When it does occur, each case should be considered most carefully on its own merits and, as ever, consultation should be considered with colleagues, with legal advisers within the defence societies, and with the British Medical Association. Careful record-keeping and good clinical practice will be the bed-rock of effective communication with patients.

6 Assessing parenting capacity

A child and adolescent psychiatrist's opinion may be sought when a child's development or behaviour is abnormal and the court wants to know to what extent parental practices are responsible for the situation. When a child is not showing any abnormality at present there may be concern that a parent will be unfit to continue to care for a child or to receive a child who has been in the care of others. Child and adolescent psychiatrists may be able to make a special contribution in the following situations:

physical abuse
psychological trauma
sexual abuse
Munchausen's syndrome by proxy/factitious illness
neglect
cruelty
emotional abuse/rejection
abandonment
gross emotional or behavioural disturbance in the child
gross developmental delay in the child
failure to thrive
deprivation
parental mental illness
parental personality disorder/eccentricity
parental addiction
parental learning disability
parental lifestyle (prostitution, multiple caretakers, homosexuality)
parental competence to care and protect
divorce proceedings
placement decisions when the child is already in alternative care
domestic violence.

Assessment will vary according to the presenting problem and only general principles are discussed. A comprehensive textbook has been published (Reder & Lucey, 1995).

Within the framework of the Children Act 1989 it is important to discuss whether any significant harm done to the child is attributable to parental acts or omissions and whether the parent is acting as a 'reasonable parent' for the child concerned. Parenting is a complex procedure taking place in complex social situations and assessment is complex also. Parenting capacity cannot be assessed simply by an interview with one parent or reference to the mental state of one parent or the other. The influence of current circumstances cannot be overemphasised. Individuals with the most unpromising backgrounds can prove themselves to be 'good enough' parents (Winnicott, 1965; Adcock & White, 1984, 1998).

The circumstances in which the question is asked are also relevant to the assessment. Very different criteria may be used in assessing the parenting capacity of a child's natural parent from that of a prospective adoptive parent (for example schizophrenia is likely to be a bar to becoming an adoptive parent but is not a sufficient reason for removing a child from a biological parent).

Parenting is rarely a function of one individual alone; thus the parenting capacity of the household may need to be assessed. Wider social supports are also relevant. The greater the social isolation of parents and the more the burden of parenting falls on one or two people, the more likely it is that parental disabilities, of whatever sort, will impinge adversely upon parenting capacity.

The child's contribution is also important. Thus at different ages children need different things from their parents. The parenting needs of a mentally- or physically-disabled young child are very different from those of a disturbed teenager. A child's temperament may also play a part in rendering him or her difficult to parent, calling for unusual qualities in the caretaker.

In court one is often dealing with value-judgements held by other people, rather than objective information about a person's ability to be a parent. Thus terms like 'mentally-retarded', 'schizophrenic', 'drug-addict', 'alcoholic', 'psychopathic', 'personality-disordered', etc., may be used to suggest that a parent is inevitably incompetent or unsuitable. The child and adolescent psychiatrist's role often may be to translate these value-laden labels into everyday language and to explain how such conditions in parents, if present, may affect children's well-being. Diagnostic labels are impressive and may carry powerful stereotyped connotations, which will be used by skilful advocates in an attempt to disqualify a parent or parents.

Assessment by child and adolescent psychiatrist or adult psychiatrist?

Complex cases may require more than one expert opinion. This is summed up by Oates (1984):

> The adult psychiatrist may see parenting in terms of its therapeutic usefulness for his patient. He may give a lower order priority to the needs of the child and to the effect of parental psychiatric and personality disorder on the child. He may be able to provide useful information on the development and aetiology of the parental condition and its course and prognosis but little in relation to parenting capacity when 'well'. The child psychiatrist may give a useful opinion on parental behaviour and attitudes and the contribution they make to the child's existing problems or risks for the future. He is more likely to be able to discuss the advantages and disadvantages of alternative care, or of one parent versus another. He will be familiar with the manifestations of minor mental illness and personality abnormalities in adults, but may not be so familiar with the implications of major adult mental illness for children and the likely cause and prognosis of such conditions.

There may be advantages in having an assessment from more than one practitioner.

Parents with learning disability

In both British and American courts, people with learning disability run a higher risk of losing their children through the action of the courts, although it is by no means established that capacity to parent successfully is related to measured intelligence.

Parenthood is rare in people with severe learning disability. No one is asserting that those who are unable to care for themselves should take sole responsibility for a dependent, defenceless baby. However, the majority of cases before the courts concern those with mild or borderline learning disability. Their limited intellectual functioning is usually recognised during their school years, but more than 90% of those found to be functioning in the mild and borderline range require no specialised services and disappear into the general population after leaving school. The women are more likely to marry than their male counterparts and they tend to do so at an earlier age than their more able female contemporaries. The Aberdeen study (Koller *et al*, 1988) following a cohort into adult life showed that women with mild disability tended to marry more able men and to take a more submissive role in the partnership. However, they were at greater risk of violence and abuse from their partners than other women. It was more difficult for them to resolve major problems and those with learning disability were found to have had poor life experiences, often with unrecognised and untreated emotional and psychiatric disorders. Their home backgrounds were more deprived and many were trying to bring up children in circumstances that even able and affluent parents would find extremely trying.

Measures of positive achievement are more helpful than standardised tests of intelligence. The advice of speech and language therapists with expertise in learning disability is helpful but too rarely available. None the less when the difficulties are appreciated and care is taken to use well-constructed plain language, lawyers have found that it is perfectly possible to obtain good instructions from a client with learning disability.

Clearly the standards to ensure the safety of a child must be the same as in any other case and a child must never be used as either a therapeutic tool or as a reward for good behaviour. But much neglect is preventable and parenting can be taught in a way that allows for a slower rate of learning, involving techniques very familiar to local learning-disability teams, without loss of dignity. Strengths can be built on and a range of supports utilised. The child's interests demand that there is good cooperation between disciplines and that the problems impeding successful parenting are accurately assessed and effectively treated. When children may not live with a birth parent, for whatever reason, information is essential and contact, direct and indirect, requires careful consideration (see Chapter 7).

Parents with psychiatric disorder

There may be advantages in having an assessment from more than one practitioner in complex cases, for example an adult psychiatrist's opinion may be sought when there is evidence of major psychiatric disorder in a parent. The child and adolescent psychiatrist should stress the implications for the child of such a disorder. If the parent needs prolonged hospitalisation, or can be expected to recover after treatment but is unfit to care for the child when ill, a report must address the child's needs for stable and continuous parenting, taking into account the child's attachment bonds and the amount and quality of parenting available while the parent is ill, including the use of those psychiatric hospitals where, when appropriate, children can be admitted with a mentally ill parent. Specialists in learning disability similarly may complement work of other clinicians.

If serious injury has been done to a child, a report by an adult forensic psychiatrist assessing the 'dangerousness' of the parent is potentially helpful.

Assessment procedure: principles to be considered

(a) Reports, verbal or written, from professional people dealing with the children and parents over time are essential. A psychiatric assessment takes place over a short time span, and must be supplemented by the longer-term observations of teachers, nursery teachers, health visitor, social worker, adult psychiatrists and others.

(b) Parents should be interviewed together, separately and with the children. Parenting skills may be tested, for example by asking one or both parents to leave the room to see whether and how they prepare the children and observing the behaviour of all parties during the brief separation. The parent(s) may be asked to perform simple child-care tasks and to play with their children (for example, "read a story to him", "draw a picture together", "can you help Johnny with this jigsaw?", and so on). The parents could be asked to plan and carry out an activity with their child while the psychiatrist observes behind a one-way screen (Jenner, 1992).

(c) If parents are not living together or not living with the children (who may be in care), it is still important for the psychiatrist to see how they behave together, if they have contact. Parents who are reasonable apart may be quite destructive together and be unable to protect the children from their hostilities.

(d) It is important that all psychiatric interviews, even for assessment purposes, should be therapeutic and should help those involved to feel 'less bad' about what is happening, if possible. The use of positive statements and genuine empathy for a parent who cares about but cannot care for a child can help that parent to accept a recommendation which is painful. Children also need help with anger and self-blame concerning their parents.

(e) The parents' relationships with other adults must be assessed. This includes grandparents, social workers, neighbours, friends, etc. A single parent living with a supportive grandparent may be able to care for a child while another, lacking this support, may not. A parent who likes and trusts a social worker may cope better than one who is suspicious and hostile.

(f) The interaction of genetic and environmental influences should be considered. For example a child with a high genetic loading for schizophrenia may need to be reared in a more stable environment than is required by a child with a lower genetic predisposition (Nuechterlein, 1986).

(g) Mentally ill or personality-disordered parents who are injurious or neglectful or who involve their children in their delusional activity are unlikely to offer competent future parenting.

(h) The duration of the parent's mental illness should be considered in relation to the age of the child. If a parent is likely to recover in six months, an older child may be fostered, but six months' fostering for a one-year-old will involve making another set of attachments and suffering if these are disturbed.

(i) Homosexual parents appear to be able to rear children satisfactorily (Kirkpatrick *et al*, 1981; Golombek *et al*, 1983).

(j) A parent may sometimes be aware of the need to give up a child for the child's sake but be fearful of family or community condemnation if this is done. These pressures need skilful exploration and, if present, need comment, with recommendations for dealing with them.

(k) Some children can be reared by disabled parents but others may have special needs which they cannot meet. The child's compatibility with the parents must be assessed in each case.

(l) Assessment of the family in their own home should be considered.

Recommendations

The psychiatrist in formulating recommendations should follow the general principles outlined in Chapter 2. In addition the following points must be considered.

(a) In recommending a temporary placement, pending the outcome of treatment for a mentally ill parent, the report should consider the effect on the child of the new attachments he or she will make, and on foster carers of rearing a child whose future with them is uncertain.

(b) In any conflict between the needs of the child and the parent, the child's needs should be afforded greater prominence. The possibility that the mental state of the parent will worsen if a child is removed or not returned must be recognised and discussed.

(c) If an opinion is formed that a parent is permanently unable to care for a child and there is no other suitable parent or relative, a legally secure future for the child is the first priority.

(d) Even if psychiatric treatment of the parent, or the passage of time, brings improvement, a child may be in need of immediate secure parenting and be unable to wait for such changes. It may be appropriate then for the psychiatrist to express an uncompromising opinion to this effect.

If treatment of parent and/or family is desirable, their willingness to undergo it and its availability must be ascertained before it is recommended.

7 Parental responsibility, residence and contact

Parental responsibility

Parental responsibility in law is conferred on both parents if married to each other at the time of the child's birth or if the child is legitimised subsequently, in accordance with the Legitimacy Act 1976, by the marriage of the parents; the Children Act 1989, section 2 and the Family Law Reform Act 1987, section 1 are also relevant. Otherwise, parental responsibility is conferred on the mother alone. This term embraces all the powers and duties of parents and guardians of a child's person and the child's estate as recognised in common law. A father who is not married to the mother (Children Act, section 4) may acquire parental responsibility, by formal agreement with her or by application to a court. It is usual for the court to grant it if the father can establish that the child is his, even if it is opposed by other parties or the parents are separated. (The status of unmarried fathers is under review. Current case law suggests a need for demonstrated commitment (Re *H* [1991] Fam 151) but the Government is considering introducing automatic parental responsibility for fathers, and this is discussed in a recent White Paper.)

Section 87 of the 1987 White Paper that preceded the Children Act 1989 stated:

> The Government accepts widespread criticism of current care law as confusing, unnecessarily complex and in places unjust. It is hard for parents and children who may be affected by it to understand its implications for them and how their rights and responsibilities may be affected. It is difficult also for professionals who must use or act in accordance with the law – social workers, lawyers, police and others. Changes are needed to rationalise, clarify and where

possible simplify the law, above all in the interests of children whose
well-being is the primary objective of child care law.

Formerly, in relation to divorce law and its effects upon children,
different tiers of court had different powers, being able to allocate
'custody', 'care and control', and 'access' as they thought appropriate.
The possibility of making orders in favour of other interested
parties, such as grandparents or step-parents, also varied widely.
There was confusion as to the difference between 'sole custody',
usually given to the mother, and 'joint custody' since one important
decision (*Dipper* v. *Dipper* (1981), FLR 31) made the point that a 'sole
custody' order did not mean that the non-custodial parent had no
rights to be consulted about the future of the child concerned, yet
the non-custodial parent could not veto long-term plans. Thus
inconsistent law was applied in an inconsistent way, with wide
variation between one court and another.

The term 'residence order' has replaced 'custody', and 'contact'
replaces 'access'. The orders available under the Act are discussed
in Chapter 13.

Separation or divorce ends the parents' personal relationship,
but their parental responsibility continues while they have dependent
children. It is obviously desirable for the children that parents find
a way of continuing a cooperative relationship. In the USA the use
of joint orders has increased and, in the UK, the Booth Committee
suggested that joint custody often would be the desirable arrangement
(Booth, 1983). There is evidence that, even when joint custody was
imposed by the courts on unwilling parents, there were fewer
disputes than with sole custody (Ilfield *et al*, 1982). Flexible use of
the new orders, or not making an order at all, may offer comparable
benefits. Although the term 'joint custody' is not now used, shared
parenting within the framework of the Children Act 1989 is a
comparable concept.

However, English courts have expressed disapproval of alternating
care and control (*R* v. *R* [1986] 150 JP 439 CA). Wherever the child
lives as the result of a residence order, he or she has to maintain
social and neighbourhood links, and attend school. In the USA and
Australia there has been a move towards shared or alternating care
and control arrangements – the child living for a part of the
week or year with each parent (Arbanel, 1979), but longer term
evaluation is lacking. In New Zealand, family law allows a 'breathing
space' for a child's family to work out a care plan before local
authority intervention. Sometimes the parent moves to where the
child is living; more often the child moves; for success, it is likely
that the parental relationship has to be reasonably harmonious and

cooperative. They must live near enough for the children to have access to one school, set of friends and leisure activities, and a satisfactory method of resolving conflicts should have been agreed.

Conflicts about residence and contact can occur between separated or divorced parents and, when care orders have been made, between parents and local authority social services departments.

Parental conflicts

The child and adolescent psychiatrist may be consulted in a residence dispute by one parent's solicitor or the court, by the Official Solicitor, or guardian ad litem. Psychiatrists also may be consulted by a divorce court welfare officer. A routine clinical referral may not mention a residence or contact dispute but this may become an issue (for the parents or the psychiatric team) during the course of assessment or therapy. The psychiatrist should adhere to principles defined in earlier chapters in regard to seeing both parents from the beginning of work with a family, wherever possible. Permission should be sought to contact solicitors to all the parties concerned and to provide a report giving an opinion on the 'least detrimental' solution for the child or children (see Goldstein *et al*, 1980*a*). This can be the basis for negotiation or, if that fails, litigation.

Either parent may be able to meet a child's basic needs for food, clothing and shelter, and less quantifiable needs for affection, continuity of care, discipline, education and the facilitation of autonomy. It may be necessary for a psychiatrist to give an opinion that this is so and, wherever possible, to help both parents continue the task of parenting. Even though the marriage is over they can pay due attention to basic child-care principles.

However, on occasion there may be clear indications that one parent offers more appropriate and consistent care than does the other and for a recommendation to this effect. It is appropriate for a psychiatrist to consider all the factors outlined in the next chapter and, in making recommendations about residence, to append an opinion about contact by the other parent and, where appropriate, other key figures such as grandparents.

Conflicts with local authorities

These may occur when a local authority is joined as a party in divorce proceedings, which may happen when child protection is at issue, in contested care applications, or when applications for revocation of care orders are opposed. In these cases it is valuable that the psychiatrist interview the social worker and foster-carers (or children's home staff) as well as the child and family. A local child and adolescent psychiatrist may recommend that an outside psychiatric opinion be sought (see Chapter 1).

The task is to have regard to legal requirements, to consider the child's best interests and to advise on the course which meets the child's needs. Rather than merely recommending a care order, or that the child returns to a parent, a psychiatrist should consider what care the child needs under this order or what supervision may be appropriate and consult the local authority as to whether it agrees with this opinion. This may, at times, mean having to point out deficiencies in the social services provision of care. Limitations in resources and training, often recognised by the authority concerned, may increase a child's difficulties. It is the advantage of independence and professional status that psychiatrists can comment on such matters and on the lack of availability of psychiatric resources.

Sometimes contact by natural parents becomes eroded before court hearings are held with regard to residence or freeing for adoption. The result may be that the child puts down roots elsewhere and, whether or not the original decision was justified, parents who have no continuing relationship with their child are disadvantaged in hearings subsequent to that decision. At such hearings the current best interests of the child, for the maintenance of the security of any new relationships, may be in conflict with those of the parents, who have wished for continued contact and that the child should return to their care.

It may be necessary for a psychiatrist to point out earlier poor decision-making and to consider whether it is still feasible or desirable to restore the child to the natural parents and, if so, to outline the best procedure for achieving it, and recommend a time-scale. Natural justice for the parents may conflict with what is in the best interests of the child.

Where parents are divorcing or separating their children are likely to experience some emotional trauma. Parents will benefit from counselling, perhaps involving mediation, on matters relating to property and finance as well as children. Under the Family Law Act 1996 they may be required to receive such a service before being eligible for legal aid. At the time of writing pilot studies are being undertaken.

If a parent is experiencing domestic violence orders may be available under the Family Law Act 1996, to provide for 'non-molestation orders' or 'occupation orders' regulating the occupation of the matrimonial home. Orders may also be available under the Protection from Harassment Act 1997.

Contact

When divorcing or separated parents cannot agree on the frequency and duration of contact visits for children with the non-resident parent, they can apply to the court for a defined contact order: Children Act, section 8. Also, a local authority has to seek a court order to terminate contact between a parent and a child subject to a care order: Children Act, section 34.

Most research on the psychological effects on children of parental separation has found that they do best when they have regular contact with the non-resident parent (Heatherington *et al*, 1979; Wallerstein & Kelly, 1980; Lund, 1984; Walczak, 1984; Mitchell, 1985, 1988), although violence from one parent to another may preclude safe contact arrangements. The Children Act 1989 takes account of this work. Children develop attachments to people with whom they have frequent, significant and mutually satisfying contact. Young children, given the opportunity, form attachments to both their parents, and often to siblings, grandparents and other close relatives, and to any other adults in the household. When parents separate, some of these attachments are disrupted to a greater or lesser degree. This occurs also when children are removed from their parents by the order of a court. Older children and adolescents usually are able to maintain contact with a parent with whom they do not live; young children are dependent on adults to make arrangements on their behalf.

About one-third to one-half of non-resident (formerly non-custodial) parents do not maintain regular contact (Murch, 1980; Maidment, 1984). Reasons given include breakdown in communication and continuing discord, violence or threats of violence, although some non-resident parents appear to believe their children would be better off without them (see Burgoyne *et al* (1987) for a fuller discussion).

Contact may be used by the resident parent as a weapon in a financial battle, and is sometimes equated with maintenance payments so that, for example, a non-resident father may refuse maintenance if he does not have contact, or a resident mother may refuse contact if payments are in default. Attempts to deal separately with maintenance with the Child Support Agency have not defused such conflicts. Children may be used as pawns in these battles and develop symptoms related to conflicting loyalties. Disputes over contact are often prolonged, taking up much legal time.

Matters to be considered in preparing a report

Advantages of contact

    (a) Contact may maintain worthwhile relationships and attachments.

    (b) Contact may help to prevent children from blaming themselves for the breakdown of the family, and reduce or prevent the formation of unhelpful and unrealistic fantasies about people with whom a child no longer lives. If supervised, it may enable children to see relatives in a different light. For example a drunken, battering father may be presented to the child at a time when the father is sober and when the child is protected.

    (c) Contact is one way of keeping children informed about the families from which they originate.

    (d) Contact is one way of helping children keep in touch with their culture of origin.

    (e) Contact is one way of informing children about a mentally or physically ill parent who is no longer able to cope with their care. It may be particularly important for a child to see a parent during a terminal illness.

    (f) Contact can be an essential component in ensuring a less difficult transition for children moving from one situation to another. For instance, children moving from one foster home to another need to meet the new people before moving, and to reassure themselves about the previous family after they have moved.

    (g) Contact is an essential part of any plan to rehabilitate children with their own families.

The same factors should be considered in relation to contact with other relatives such as grandparents and siblings. Contact between siblings who have been together through a series of changes and adversities may be of particular value and importance to a child.

In principle, contact should be the right of the child. In practice, many difficulties may make regular contact impossible to achieve or contact may not be in the child's best interests.

    (a) The resident, foster or adoptive parent may feel threatened by contact visits, fearing to lose the child. This anxiety can be sensed by the child who may develop behavioural difficulties in relation to the contact visits which are then used as evidence that these are harmful.

    (b) The resident parent may become depressed or otherwise disturbed by the visits. This then might affect their care of the child, who then may develop symptoms.

(c) Either parent may use the child in his or her battle with the other parent. The child may become the sole means of communication between them.

(d) A parent may use contact as a way of attempting to restore a relationship undesired by the other parent, to reduce the guilt felt about being a bad parent, or to control a former partner.

(e) A non-resident father may never have lived with his child, for example when the marriage ended before the birth of the child. The frequency of contact needed in order to establish a relationship would be much greater than that needed to maintain it. If the child is very young such frequent visits may be impractical or undesirable, given the overwhelming need to establish a secure relationship between the baby and the primary caretaker.

(f) An altruistic father may feel that his young child might be confused by having to relate to two fathers (when a step-parent appears) and may, unless counselled, decide to drop out of the picture, or a mother may push for his disappearance for the same reason.

(g) Because of their loyalty to those having their day-to-day care, children may avoid talking about non-resident parents or other relatives. It is sometimes deduced from such behaviour by parents and others that children have no interest in contact and could derive no benefit from it. Children may also play one parent off against the other, reporting to one discomforting information about the other, especially if it seems of interest to the recipient.

(h) A child may resist seeing a non-resident parent if he or she has been badly treated or abused by that parent or if the child is aware that the parent has committed serious crimes such as murder or rape. A child may need protection from continuing threats of violence to the resident parent (as may the parent).

The role of the child and adolescent psychiatrist in advising about contact

Child and adolescent psychiatrists may be consulted by social services, the court, divorce court welfare officers, guardians ad litem, or parents, foster parents and grandparents and their solicitors about the desirability of contact, how frequent it should be and of what duration. Psychiatrists are often asked to support the view that contact with one parent is harmful. If contact is not an agreed, harmonious part of a child's life, that child is likely to be excited and anxious before, during and after contact visits. Stopping or reducing contact may indeed end aggression against the resident parent, nightmares or soiling. However, abrupt termination of the child's relationship with a parent may not be helpful in the longer term, and the psychiatrist must consider and discuss such issues as these.

The views of all relevant adults should be sought and considered. These may include foster parents, social workers, siblings and other relatives. The wishes of children should be ascertained, while making it clear to them it is only adults who can make decisions. Clearly, the older and more mature the child, the greater is the importance attached to the child's views.

The child and adolescent psychiatrist should bear in mind the right of the child to contact with parents and extended family and the right to maintain significant attachments and relationships. The psychiatrist will have to evaluate in each case the advantages and disadvantages for each child, when there is serious conflict between the parents. It is necessary to achieve a position which helps others involved in the case to discriminate between those factors that create temporary disturbance in the children and those factors that are likely to cause permanent damage to their emotional development.

Disputing parents should always be asked about the disposal of the property of the marriage. Unresolved arguments about money and property frequently underlie disputes over residence and contact. Expert mediation may be necessary for the parents (Parkinson, 1986) before contact can be established. Its availability should be discussed with them. Where appropriate, a psychiatrist may recommend a therapeutic programme to assist parents and others to understand the causes of the child's behaviour and help contact become less troublesome.

Where the parents separated before the birth, the psychiatrist needs to be satisfied that the advantage to the child in establishing this new relationship outweighs the disadvantages. It may be better to advise a non-resident parent to postpone contact visits until the child is older, keeping in touch through cards and birthday presents and/or providing maintenance (the importance of maintenance is psychological as well as practical). A resident parent who feels unthreatened may be better able to accept a legitimate request for contact later when it will indeed be of direct benefit to the child.

At times, frequent contact may be granted by a department of social services and endorsed by courts out of compassion for a parent deprived of a child. The psychiatrist must consider whether the frequency is in the best interests of the child, given that residence may never be restored.

Lawyers may need help in distinguishing the signs of short-term disturbance occurring in children who probably are very upset, showing a healthy reaction to upheaval, from longer-term or pathological dysfunction. The former may require therapeutic help rather than termination of contact; the latter may not improve while visits continue.

The report

This should lead to a clear statement of the relevant advantages and disadvantages of continuing or terminating contact and the psychiatrist's views as to which course in the long term will be less harmful to the child. The reasons for contact, its frequency and its purpose should be addressed.

A report should point out possible practical problems and how these might be overcome. It may state that contact conflicts are not likely to be resolved until the parents have resolved other conflicts such as those over housing or money. On occasion, referral of the parents to a mediation service may be recommended.

In describing the details of a contact programme, the age and maturity of any children involved are obviously important and appropriate comment should be made. For example, babies should not be subjected to orders that strain their attachment to the caretaking parent. Toddlers are probably too young to stay overnight with a non-resident parent with whom they have never lived and some children may not tolerate overnight stays before the age of six years. Recommendations should complement those of court officers responsible for assessing accommodation and other practical details that also may require comment. Thus, in principle, the more contact is a routine part of life, the less the risk that visits become a treat when compared to daily life with a resident parent. It may be helpful for visits to take place in a neutral setting such as with a mutual friend, or with a grandparent who is respected by both parties. A contact centre run by a local authority or a voluntary organisation may be suitable. Contact after prolonged breaks requires special care – for example a series of brief visits may be appropriate, before arranging a weekend stay or holiday.

The psychiatrist, if commenting on a suggested programme, needs to bear in mind the purpose of contact. This may be for the continuation of a worthwhile relationship, to reassure the child, to provide him or her with information about people formerly important to him, or as a preliminary to possible rehabilitation of the child to the family. Where a child is freed for adoption there may be a need for visits from former family members before and after the placement in the permanent family. Some adoptive parents are now prepared to allow continuing contact with key members of the former family. The need regularly to review the progress of any programme should be emphasised in a report to the court concerned.

Child abduction   Richard White

Within the framework of the Children Act 1989, disputes between parents about the exercise of parental responsibility are regulated by section 8 orders. If a parent removes a child from the other parent in defiance of a section 8 Residence Order, it is not a criminal offence but it may be a contempt of court for which the court may impose a fine or imprisonment. In order to enforce return of the child, it is necessary to obtain an order from the court authorising a court officer or a police officer to take charge of the child and to deliver him or her to the person who should be caring for the child.

Different countries of the UK have different court systems. Where an order is in force in one part of the UK, it will be recognised and can be enforced in another.

Removal from the UK

Prevention is better than cure! It is easier to stop a child leaving the country than getting a child back who has been taken abroad. Once he has left the country it is more difficult to discover his whereabouts and once the child is found, the foreign country may not order his return. There are a number of ways in which removal can be made more difficult. The court may make a section 8 Prohibited Steps Order. The Port Stop procedure may be invoked, involving notification to the police if removal is believed to be imminent and the point of departure is known. The court may make an order authorising publicity to help trace a missing child. Any person who might have information about the whereabouts of the child can be ordered to appear before the court to give evidence. An order may be made for the surrender of a passport or the UK Passport Agency may be asked not to issue it. Prevention has been made more difficult because of the relaxation of passport checks at border controls.

Because removal from the country without consent is a criminal offence, it is also a crime to attempt to remove a child. If the police are alerted to a threat of removal, they can notify likely ports of departure that a child might be abducted. The abducting parent will then be turned back if they attempt to leave with the child and in some cases might be arrested. No court order is required.

A parent or guardian of a child under 16, or a person in whose favour a Residence Order is in force in respect of the child, commits a criminal offence if they take the child out of the UK without the consent of each person who has parental responsibility for the child. No offence is committed if the person believes that consent has been or would be given or is being unreasonably withheld, but if consent is refused it is a wise precaution to obtain the consent of the court. A person having a Residence Order may take or send the child out of the country for up to a month, provided there is no order in force prohibiting removal. In practice, anyone taking a child out of the country for any period of time would be well advised to ensure that they have the consent of every person having parental responsibility.

If a child is taken from this country or brought to this country by a parent against the wishes of the other parent, the courts will seek to assist the wronged parent by returning the children immediately without consideration of the merits. The steps to take will depend on the country from which the child has been removed, the country to which he is removed and the circumstances of the removal.

Under the terms of the Hague or European Conventions, the country to which a child has been wrongfully removed should seek to return the child, usually without consideration of the merits, to the country from which he has been removed, where any dispute about the child should be resolved. The purpose of the Conventions is to ensure the prompt return of the child and to discourage unlawful removal. The Hague Convention, to which many countries worldwide are signatories, applies to children under 16, who have been removed or retained in breach of the rights of a parent. It is not necessary for there to be a court order in force. The European Convention applies only where there is a breach of an existing order.

If a child is wrongfully removed from the UK, in England and Wales assistance should be sought from the Child Abduction Unit of the Lord Chancellor's Department. This is the 'Central Authority' which deals with such cases. If the country to which the child has been removed is a Convention country, the unit will contact the corresponding central authority in that country.

If the child has been taken to a non-Convention country, a parent may seek a court order for the return of the child, through a section 8 Specific Issue or Prohibited Steps Order, or through wardship. There are likely to be difficulties in enforcing the order abroad. If the abducting parent has property in this country which could be sequestered, it may be possible to persuade that parent to return the child. Without that lever the wronged parent may have no alternative to seeking to obtain an order for return from a court in the foreign country, after consideration of the merits of the case.

Removal to the UK

If a child is wrongfully brought to this country, the parent from whom the child has been removed can approach their central authority, which will contact the central authority in this country. The authority will instruct a solicitor in private practice, selected from an approved panel. The parent is entitled to free legal aid. The solicitor will make an application in the High Court for the immediate return of the child.

If the country from which the child has been removed is a non-Convention country, the parent from whom the child has been removed may take proceedings in this country by way of application for a section 8 order or through wardship. The court is likely to apply the principles established in the Conventions, and unless there are persuasive reasons for not doing so, will order immediate return.

Check-list

(a) Is the conflict between parents alone or between parents and a local authority?

(b) What is the legal status of the child?

(c) Who is asking for an opinion (e.g. legal representative of parent, legal representative of child, court officer, Official Solicitor)?

(d) Obtain permission from the court, where necessary, for interviewing the child.

(e) Formulate an opinion about the least detrimental solution for the child with regard to residence.

(f) Having arrived at this, form an opinion as to the best interests of the child regarding contact, direct and/or indirect, with non-resident parents and other key relatives.

(g) In preparing your report, consider your role as an 'independent' or 'local' psychiatrist.

(h) Follow the check-list in Chapter 2.

8   Child abuse and neglect

This chapter deals mainly with principles relevant specifically to the preparation of court reports relating to child abuse and neglect. The bibliography includes extensive clinical and research references, which are essential reading.

Subsequent to the work of Kempe in the early 1960s (see Kempe & Helfer, 1987), doctors increasingly have become aware of the high prevalence of child abuse, the many ways it can present and its long-lasting effects. Child abuse, perhaps more than any other issue, has led to a greater willingness by doctors to work in partnership with employees of education and social services departments and with lawyers. The General Medical Council (1987) expressed the view that if a doctor believes a child is being physically or sexually abused, it is his duty to disclose this information to a third party. Initially, the role of the child and adolescent psychiatrist was relatively peripheral. The lead in diagnostic issues and in preparing evidence for the court was taken by paediatricians. Psychiatric intervention might arise after court proceedings had been completed, to help social workers make appropriate plans for the long-term future of the abused child.

The concept of child abuse has widened considerably. Clinical work has demonstrated that the fractured arm of an abused child might heal relatively rapidly, but the damage caused by accompanying emotional abuse might continue for many years. Sexual abuse has leapt into prominence and there has been growing acknowledgement that emotional abuse accompanies direct physical and sexual abuse but also occurs without it, and must always be considered. The role of the child and adolescent psychiatrist has become more central in terms of diagnosis, treatment and the preparation of evidence for court hearings.

The Children Act 1989 continued this process by defining 'significant harm' – the criteria for a care order in terms of 'harm' cover physical, sexual and emotional maltreatment, or impairment of physical or mental health or developmental problems attributable to the failure of parents to give appropriate care.

It is customary to divide abuse into physical injury, neglect, emotional ill-treatment, sexual abuse and 'grave concern' (Department of Health and Social Security, 1988 *a,b,c*). Such categories are not mutually exclusive. For example, sexual abuse almost by definition must include emotional ill-treatment and neglect. Failure to thrive merges imperceptibly with physical abuse.

Each of these categories of abuse has a formal definition, and severe cases of any type will present few problems of recognition. However, the dividing line between extreme variations of normal parenting and actual abuse lies within a grey area which is difficult to define (see Adcock & White, 1998).

In describing the effects of continuing abuse on a child's psychological functioning, psychiatrists can make a major contribution. They often will be asked to give an opinion as to how the needs of an abused child may best be met. This role should be wider than making individual responses to requests from a party to a legal hearing. The child and adolescent psychiatrist should be familiar with, and be involved with, the administrative framework of area child protection committees, and child protection procedures, in any district. (See Young (1987), Butler-Sloss (1988) and Bazell (1989) for a detailed description of this and of the legal aspects of child abuse.) The Department of Health (1991*a,b*; 1994*a*) has provided guidelines on inter-agency cooperation in assessing and protecting abused and neglected children. As they appear, subsequent guidelines should be retained in departmental libraries.

The role of the child and adolescent psychiatrist in court proceedings

Before being involved in any abuse case, it is important for the child and adolescent psychiatrist to define what can and cannot be done. Psychiatrists can determine whether emotional abuse has been, or is, occurring. They can describe a child's mental state and emotional development and give an opinion as to whether emotional abuse or neglect may be causal to any pathology seen. They can comment on the quality of family relationships, the emotional responsiveness and child-rearing skills of the parents, and on whether the child's state is attributable to parenting failures.

In addition, however, there will be various issues particularly relevant to abuse which can and should always be considered. One major issue is the investigation which will take place when child abuse is suspected. In addition to diagnostic assessments and medical examinations, there may, for criminal proceedings, be interviews by the police, the gathering of evidence by the child's guardian ad litem and solicitor and by experts appointed by parents and other parties. The psychiatrist must be prepared to comment on the effect on the child of these different investigations and endeavour to prevent repeated interviews if it is felt that they will be detrimental.

When sexual abuse is alleged some workers have used emotionally 'invasive' techniques whose reliability and validity is as yet uncertain and which may be abusive in unskilled hands (Butler-Sloss, 1988). The advantages and the potential harm of these techniques may require comment (Royal College of Psychiatrists, 1988). At times a child will, for reasons of protection, have to be removed urgently from the home, possibly with police accompanying social workers. At other times the same procedure is used when the urgency is less obvious. This may require comment. The requirements to be satisfied in the Child Protection Order and the Child Assessment Order make removal from home subject to challenge, and therefore fewer children are likely to be removed arbitrarily. (A Department of Health circular (1995) outlines principles of good practice for social workers and police.)

Major questions asked of a psychiatrist may concern the relative advantages and disadvantages of separating a child from the parents and of placing him or her in the care of a local authority; for example, under the Children Act 1989, the court must be convinced that, despite 'significant harm', the alternative to remaining at home is to the child's advantage. The psychiatrist's view of the parents' willingness or ability to provide a better standard of parenting is most relevant (see Chapter 9) in the context of the 'welfare check-list' that the court has to consider in each case. The court has to consider the needs of the particular child, and the child and adolescent psychiatrist may well have relevant views on this.

Boundaries of the psychiatrist's role

Psychiatric and psychological factors are only two strands among the many to be considered in any case of alleged child abuse. Problems arise when a psychiatric examination in a clinic shows well-functioning children, and warm devoted parents, but outside reports point to other failures of parenting. An example was seen in a family with two active toddlers. On examination there was clearly joy and warmth between all the family members. The children, although slightly delayed in development, showed no gross psychiatric disorders. Unfortunately, the parents' lifestyle led them rarely to get out of bed before 11.00. The children could make their way out of the front door of their flat, and two near-fatal accidents had occurred. Despite a great deal of practical advice and help and protestations that things would improve, the children remained at risk. The referring social worker was unhappy with the psychiatric assessment. It had to be pointed out that although in this case there were no psychiatric grounds for a care order, there were very powerful and obvious social ones. Emotional warmth would be of no use to a dead child. This type of situation is one where a major task of the child and adolescent psychiatrist is to explain the importance of practical and social work observations such as that the parents are not willing or able to provide appropriate care.

This caution clearly applies to many cases of physical and sexual abuse, as with the learning-disabled mother, who obviously loves her child but whose rough handling has caused many fractures and who may not be 'able' to provide care. Here it is safety, not psychology, which is the point at issue. The child and adolescent psychiatrist must not attempt to take on the role of 'expert' in such areas as physical safety or adequate diet, unless he or she really does have special knowledge and expertise in these fields. It is a misuse of the role of expert witness to present what is basically a common-sense opinion on a topic unrelated to one's area of expertise.

The assessment of parenting (see Chapter 6), and of willingness or capacity to change it, involves weighing up information and observations from many sources, and the child and adolescent psychiatrist may be useful in providing a report which helps the court to evaluate and attach weight to the various parts of the evidence. If there is clear medical evidence for physical or sexual abuse, there must be no attempt to confirm or refute that evidence by the psychiatrist. The question to be answered is whether the psychiatric findings are important in their own right and whether they are consistent with those provided by other experts (see Reder & Lucey, 1995).

In cases of severe abuse, criminal proceedings against a parent may be taking place concurrently with the care hearing. It is not the task of a child and adolescent psychiatrist to help to obtain the conviction of a perpetrator of abuse, but to protect the child. There will be times when there is insufficient evidence to convict a parent, but sufficient to justify removing the children. It should be noted, however, that in certain circumstances, information obtained by a psychiatrist in the course of his or her duties might be required as factual evidence in the criminal proceedings against a parent. There is also the possibility that psychiatric evidence may be called to refute the evidence of the child.

Emotional abuse

Here the child and adolescent psychiatrist can give a true expert opinion as to whether abuse is occurring or has occurred, the likely outcome for the child if nothing changes, and how the child's situation may be improved. It would be reassuring to be able to draw a line beyond which emotional abuse could be said to have reached a level so unacceptable that a care order might be justified on psychiatric grounds, but this, alas, is not the case, and each particular problem must be assessed on its own merits.

It is useful, however, to consider two components which, if present, may lead the psychiatrist to feel on firm ground in diagnosing emotional abuse (Royal College of Psychiatrists, 1982). The first is a persistent pattern of parental behaviour which appears unrelated to the needs of the child. The second is the presence of severe emotional or behavioural problems in that child. The combination is important. One sees parents whose lifestyle appears eccentric and quite inappropriate. If, however, their children are developing well and show no significant delays or deviations, it is inappropriate to speak of abuse. One might disapprove of a particular lifestyle, but that is not a psychiatric matter.

Equally, the presence of gross behavioural problems in a child, in the absence of obvious parental deviation, should not be taken as grounds for speaking of emotional abuse. Child temperamental and genetic factors, or other environmental ones, may be important causative factors. The appropriate response to a situation like this is to offer help and treatment. The failure of parents to take up offers of treatment for a child with a socially disabling symptom, such as encopresis or an anxiety-provoking illness such as asthma or epilepsy, could, however, be seen as grounds for speaking of emotional abuse, or at least as showing that the child's mental or physical health or development was being impaired through parental failure to provide care.

Emotional abuse is specifically a psychiatric matter, yet difficult to define. Three examples are given below; in each case the psychiatric team considered referral to the appropriate department of social services.

(a) A girl of seven was referred at the request of her head teacher. When questioned by teachers the child insisted she was a boy. Her mother was convinced that her daughter had been changed temporarily by a spell cast by her mother-in-law. The mother's belief was explicable in cultural terms but follow-up was offered because the child was confused and withdrawn and had no friends. Appointments were not kept.

(b) A boy of six was referred to a day unit because of bizarre behaviour at school. He would drink from puddles, eat from dustbins, and roll in dirt. He had not started to read or write. He was of normal intelligence and showed no evidence of psychosis. He was grossly overweight to a point of being extremely physically clumsy. His clothes and body smelt of faeces and urine. He was called 'smelly Bill' or 'Fatty' by other children, who shunned him. His behaviour was seen as an expression of his very low self-esteem. His parents lived in remarkable squalor, and they too smelled equally bad. They could see no problem at all with their child, or with their own parental standards.

(c) A 14-year-old boy of normal intelligence had always soiled. He was isolated and bullied at school. His attainments were poor. He had no interests outside his home. He had never been to a cinema or any form of sporting activity. His mother would bathe him each day when he returned from school. For one week she had cooperated with the psychologist, who set up a programme of behavioural therapy, but then she stopped it because she found it 'silly'.

In each case there was parenting which did not meet the needs of the child who then showed mental ill health or developmental disability. There was an inability or unwillingness by the parents to use treatment. In cases such as these it is not easy for the psychiatrist to give a firm recommendation such as that the child might be removed permanently from a family. Rather, the psychiatrist should be able to spell out the likely consequences to the child of either remaining in an unchanging situation or of moving to a new one. Montgomery (1989) discusses the relevant legal and evidential issues with reference to the possible use of the powers offered by the Children Act 1989. Speight (1989) covers clinical issues, for example the use of a supervision order with requirements for psychiatric treatment or parental counselling.

Sexual abuse

Because the sexual abuse of children causes such profound emotional reactions among both the general public and professionals, there has been a tendency for it to be seen as essentially different from other forms of abuse. Specialised interviewing techniques have been developed to detect it.

There is considerable controversy over the role of the child psychiatrist in its assessment and management. In terms of the effects of sexual abuse there is little disagreement. If a child is suffering a psychiatric disorder caused by the abuse and by associated factors, such as accompanying abnormal family relationships, treatment by a child and adolescent psychiatrist obviously is appropriate. The role of the psychiatrist in helping rehabilitate a child back into a family, after the abuse has been acknowledged and stopped, is accepted.

The controversy is over the assessment of abuse (Royal College of Psychiatrists, 1988; Smith & Bentovim, 1994). Most child and adolescent psychiatrists would see their role here as being in general very similar to that of any other referral, that is, determining whether a psychiatric disorder is present and if so what is its nature and how might the child best be helped. Sexual abuse would be seen as an aetiological factor (Kolvin *et al*, 1988). The presence of a psychiatric disorder, particularly with certain patterns of symptoms, could be used to support the possibility that sexual abuse had occurred.

Some practitioners in addition would see their role as specifically to determine whether the abuse had occurred, the extent of it, and who was the perpetrator. Techniques derived from psychiatric treatment, such as the use of sexually explicit dolls, or circular questioning, have been developed for this purpose. The controversy is whether psychiatrists, trained to assess and treat illness, can and should adapt their techniques to become investigators of alleged assaults, a role possibly best left to police or child protection social workers trained in the collection of factual information for forensic purposes. Whether or not child and adolescent psychiatrists use these techniques, they must be familiar with the literature on their use (Bentovim *et al*, 1988; Kolvin *et al*, 1988; Smith & Bentovim, 1994; Department of Health, 1988*c,d*; Department of Health and Social Security, 1995 and Brandon *et al*, 1998, provide an overview of recent work in this field) and with the arguments about their validity. They should be able to justify in court why they were or were not included in the assessment.

The concept of psychological trauma

Much has been learned about the effects on children of war, disaster and witnessing violence since the last edition of this book. Since early research focused on adults, the effects on children were underestimated, being seen through the eyes of parents, teachers and other adults, often also suffering from trauma. The need of children to be cared for and the wish of adults not to cause distress by speaking to children of their experiences meant that these remained largely unexplored. This is changing: we now learn about the effects of trauma on children by speaking to them, attending to their drawings, play and behaviour and by being with them when they re-enact or relive their experiences. ICD–10 (World Health Organization, 1992) and DSM–IV (American Psychiatric Association, 1994) now identify and classify these effects, our understanding of which is being informed by clinical work and research. Clarifying the varying effects of disasters upon children according to their age, gender, culture, and earlier and subsequent life experiences, is an important mental health task of particular value to forensic child and adolescent psychiatrists. Herman (1992) and Black *et al* (1997) provide an overview of the current field of knowledge. Pynoos and colleagues (1986, 1990, 1992) discuss interview techniques and intervention techniques in bereaved and traumatised children.

The referral

Before accepting a referral, it is important to discuss with the referrers what exactly is required. In cases of abuse the request may cover one of the following points.

(a) Consultation to the referring agency. Social workers or others may require a psychiatrist's help in decision-making at a case conference, to decide whether a full assessment is necessary or whether there is sufficient evidence for them to go to court without further investigation.

(b) Child and adolescent psychiatrists may be required to assess the situation as it is at the time of referral. They may be asked to comment on the functioning of children and the parenting capacity within a family.

(c) Whether treatment is needed and whether the clinic can provide it.

(d) A type of referral to be encouraged is a request to assess both whether emotional abuse is occurring and whether change is possible. Continuing assessments of the degree of change brought about by therapeutic intervention may be a useful contribution.

Background information

Before discussing the family with other care workers it is helpful to obtain background information as already outlined in Chapter 6, viz:

(a) Social work assessment of the family background.

(b) How the family and the workers were able to implement any work offered.

(c) Medical records of parents, if appropriate.

(d) Medical records of the children, including height and weight charts.

(e) Report by health visitor, if appropriate. (In one clinic health visitors are asked to fill in a specific referral form which gives relevant background information about the family. They will also ask the parents to fill in a behavioural check-list (Richman, 1971); a diary of three days in the life of a child in the family and a sleep diary (if appropriate). This gives useful background information about the family and how they perceive their child before the family comes to the clinic.)

(f) School/nursery reports.

Full discussion with the referrers is helpful so as to ascertain their opinion of the family. This will tell something about how the referring agency sees the family and how the family may view them.

The assessment

Most child and adolescent psychiatric teams arrange to see the family together and each member separately. If a parent does not have contact with a child, he/she should initially be given an appointment separately.

The family

The assessment of the family should cover the following areas:

In parents

(a) The parents' acceptance of their responsibility and their ability to protect children from accidents and illnesses, and to provide food, shelter, education, nurturing and consistent care.

(b) The parents' background, mental state, understanding of themselves, and their understanding of the problems they have within the family; and the possibility of change and motivation for change.

(c) Relationship within the marriage.

(d) Assessment of parents' ability to act together in parenting the children.

(e) How parents solve problems and make decisions.

(f) Who disciplines and how that discipline is carried out.

(g) What family rules there are, and whether they are appropriate.

(h) From whom the family get its support (friends, family, professionals, etc.).

(i) How family members use this support.
(j) The relationships between the parents; the parents and the children; the children themselves.
(k) How they interact in the session when tasks are suggested (see Chapter 6).
(l) Whether they protect the children while in the session.
(m) Whether they relate to one child differently from the others.

If either parent has a severe psychiatric illness it might be wise to recommend a full assessment by a general or possibly a forensic psychiatrist.

In the children

The areas to be addressed are:

(a) Physical state, height and weight, coordination, any disease or disability which may require special parenting.
(b) The presence of psychiatric disorder – its nature and severity and prognosis.
(c) The child's developmental level, in particular language and social skills.
(d) The child's educational attainments.
(e) The child's relationships and attachments.

Techniques

Techniques that might be used in addition to a full interview and observation could include family trees, family games, sculpting and enactment, etc. (see Reder & Lucey (1995) for a discussion of these and related techniques). Play materials appropriate to the age of the child would be important; a child's drawings and repetitive enactments may be highly significant.

The objectives of assessment

By the end of the assessment it should be possible to give an opinion on the following:

(a) Whether abuse is happening (i.e. has significant harm occurred) and if so, to whom and by whom.
(b) What effect it is having on those exposed to it and whether it is significant.
(c) Why the abuse is happening, what factors are relevant to its causation, and the relationship to parental failure to care.
(d) What changes in the family are necessary to prevent it continuing.

(e) What work needs to be implemented to promote change, who should do it, and the willingness or ability of parents to change.

(f) If it is not possible to change the situation through a voluntary partnership, whether statutory processes (e.g. supervision or care orders) would make a difference and what contributions need to be made by professionals.

Writing the report

As in writing a report for court, whatever the underlying problems, it is important to outline the various stages in the assessment. An opinion and recommendations may be given on the lines suggested above.

The assessment of emotional or sexual abuse is particularly difficult. The report and its recommendations should be written in very clear language.

9 Placement issues

When children are known to local authority services and may be received into care, child and adolescent psychiatrists often are asked to comment upon the suitability of various placement options open to the local authority itself or to a court already concerned with the child. It is necessary to know these options and how they may affect individual children and, in giving advice, to bear in mind the issues discussed in Chapter 1 and the legal matters in Chapter 13.

Permanency planning

The concept of permanency planning emerged in the 1970s and is still applicable to all children known to a department of social services. Wherever possible the plan should be that resources are made available to enable children to remain with and thrive in their original families. If they are received into care the aim still should be to return them to the family as soon, as smoothly and as safely as possible. Only if neither of these plans is feasible should alternatives be considered. Any such alternative also should involve the establishment of a permanent home in which the child may live until he or she has grown up. Children Act 1989 guidelines uphold these principles.

These aims arose through recognition that psychological harm is done to children who 'drift' in and out of care, moving perhaps from their original family to foster carers or to children's homes. An essential part of the concept is that the time-scale within which plans are made must fit in with the child's developmental needs. For example, a 10-year-old may be able to wait a year for a permanent home, whereas a one-year-old cannot.

A psychiatrist may be asked specific questions about the individual child and family at various points of involvement with the legal and care systems; the child may be with the family of origin, subject to an emergency protection order, child assessment order, or interim care order, or there may be disputes between the natural parents and the local authority about plans to place the child away from the original family. The question of contact between the child and family (Chapter 7) must be borne in mind throughout. Child and adolescent psychiatrists may contribute when plans are in motion to place a child permanently away from the family of origin.

Factors relating to the child and family

Psychiatrists are often asked to comment on or 'measure' the child's attachment to the family of origin. It may be necessary to provide a theoretical discussion of this concept, to distinguish between secure and insecure attachments or to advise that young or emotionally immature children may be strongly attached to highly abusive parents. It may be useful to rephrase or amplify questions asked in letters of instruction, for example, "to what extent will the child be damaged if the attachment is broken" or, "to what extent can the child form new and satisfying attachments?". The psychiatrist should consider commenting on attachments additional to those between children and parents. Older siblings may play an important parental role, sibling relationships having become a source of security, particularly where parenting has become poor. There may be less strong attachments if there have been prolonged periods of separation, if children are identified with opposing factions within a conflict-ridden family or are infants. There is little research evidence concerning the effects of splitting sibships but clinical experience suggests that this is often distressing to older children and may lead to significant difficulties in maintaining a successful placement (see also Berridge & Cleaver, 1987).

These factors should be borne in mind, along with the practical difficulties in finding a single placement, particularly one intended to last until the children are grown up. In giving advice it may be necessary to balance the harmful effects of splitting a large sibship against the harmful effects of keeping the children together in an unsatisfactory or impermanent home or institution, while seeking a permanent home willing and able to take the complete sibship.

When making recommendations a child and adolescent psychiatrist may be asked to comment on whether or not a child shows psychiatric disorder which will require treatment. It is very difficult to predict the effect of placement upon commonly occurring conduct and emotional disorders, outcome being related to the quality of the home in which the child is placed rather than to the nature of the disorder (Bohman, 1981; Clarke, 1981; Lindsay, 1995). However, it may be useful to question expectations that problems of one sort or another have to be tolerated since many (e.g. enuresis, encopresis, sleep disturbance, post-traumatic stress disorder) are susceptible to appropriate psychiatric treatment (see Rutter *et al* (1994) for details of current therapeutic procedures). In preparing reports for a court it is important to give a realistic assessment of the type of treatment which may be effective and of its availability to the child.

Where there is a dispute as to whether or not a child should return to his or her own family, the psychiatrist may be asked to give an independent opinion. It is advisable to comment upon the circumstances leading to the child being removed from home, whether alternatives could be or should have been considered and whether adverse circumstances are likely to recur, if the child is now returned to the family home. It will be necessary to consider the length of time the child has been away from his or her family, what contact has taken place and, this often being controversial, the quality and intensity of social work help offered to the family and the child. There will also be a need to evaluate the current circumstances in which the child is living and the wishes and opinions of current caretakers.

The psychiatrist should consider the presence or absence of specific parental disabilities such as learning disability, personality disorder, psychiatric illness, drug addiction, etc., and, if such conditions are present, the likelihood of improvement or response to treatment and the relevant time-scale. Opinions from general and forensic psychiatrists may be necessary. An opinion should be formed regarding any possibility of change in family relationships likely to reduce conflict or violence, protect the child from abuse or neglect and facilitate his or her appropriate development.

Psychiatrists should consider the wishes of the child and the extent to which these wishes are based on age-appropriate and realistic assessment of the situation, the wishes of the parents and parent substitutes and the degree to which these are achievable. It may be necessary to offer separate interviews to each parent and to consider any attempt they might make to disguise or deny difficulties in the hope that this will lead to a 'favourable' court decision. They should also bear in mind the extent to which known risks may be mitigated by the provision of supervision and help from local services, the availability of such services and the willingness of the family to make use of them.

Regarding possible decisions available to the court, the writer of a report should be prepared to comment on criteria for assessing failure and on further decisions to be made subsequent to failure. Psychiatrists may be asked to consider the value of possible 'specific issues' and 'prohibited steps' orders (see Chapter 13, p. 107).

Resources and research

Local authorities vary in their support of the concept of permanency planning, the availability of funds and resources and in the use they make of voluntary family placement agencies such as the National Society for the Prevention of Cruelty to Children (via its treatment projects), Barnardos, National Children's Home Action for Children, British Agencies for Adoption and Fostering, Parents for Children, Catholic Children's Society, etc.

It is important therefore to talk with a child's social workers about resources available to them and to the child. For example, a local authority which arranges foster placements in an ad hoc way is less able to foster a seriously disturbed teenager than is an authority where there are 'professional' foster parents and specialist teenage fostering support schemes. A planned trial of increasing contact as a prelude to returning an abused child home probably carries less risk where the local authority is able to monitor the family's progress at a specialist family centre. Theoretically, foster services now range from short-term or emergency care to longer-term care and specialist fostering – for example, relief foster care to families with disabled children, fostering delinquent or highly disturbed teenagers for agreed periods of time and 'assessment' fostering offered in some local authorities to children in need of detailed investigation and planning from a safe temporary base. Rowe and colleagues (1983, 1989) discuss the development of fostering during the 1980s, and the Department of Health (1991*b*) offers an overview of research on placement issues.

Some local authorities maintained residential 'observation and assessment centres' where children could stay for relatively limited periods of time. Such centres sometimes provided a useful breathing space during which further information about the child and family could be gathered before decisions about long-term placement. Tutt (1981) offered a critique of these institutions and their (considerable) limitations. These institutions are now few in number and their use may discontinue although some voluntary agencies offer comparable facilities, sometimes called residential assessment centres where whole families are admitted. We know of no evaluative studies of these centres.

The psychiatrist should know something of the children's homes in the area where the child lives. The number of residential children's homes has been much reduced and numbers continue to shrink. This is partially appropriate, given the recognition that young children do very badly in institutions, but is not an adequate response to the needs of at least some older adolescents who, given they have firm links with their family of origin, may be in need of a safe place away from their family where they may complete their schooling and receive care less demanding than that available to them in a substitute family. The wishes of older children should be borne in mind. It should also be remembered however that some institutions for children suffer from high staff turnover and a child's difficulties may reflect those of an institution rather than those of the original family.

Consideration on similar lines should be given to plans to place children in residential schools. This may be useful where a family is then able to care for a child during holiday periods but is unlikely to be helpful if a child is returned from a residential school to a variety of foster homes or children's homes. Comment on such plans may be made from the specialist viewpoint of a child and adolescent psychiatrist.

Yarrow & Klein's (1980) research established that the advantage of moving to a more satisfactory environment, even for a young child, outweighs the disadvantage of a break in continuity of care. Wolkind (1994) outlines the contributions of developmental psychology and of research into alternative forms of permanency planning. The psychiatrist should know about this and related literature when consulted about plans to place a child away from a family, having due regard for current law.

Local authorities which wish to make such plans increasingly turn to child and adolescent psychiatrists to help them make preparations, evaluate the parents' ability to cooperate and advise on the time-scale appropriate to the developmental stage of the child. They, and child and adolescent psychiatrists, work in a climate where there is strong concern about the rights of birth parents and about the concept of natural justice. In one test case (Re *H*, Re *W* [1983] 4 FLR 614) where a local authority was thought by the judge to have relied substantially on the passage of time to make its case for adoption, rather than presenting evidence that persistent work had been done with the natural parents which had been unsuccessful in rehabilitating the child, adoption was refused. The Children Act 1989 strongly emphasises partnership between parents and support services for children in need, refocusing lawyers', social workers' and physicians' attention on the delicate balance between the rights of the children and the responsibilities of parents.

Freeing for adoption and adoption applications

If rehabilitation has not succeeded or is not appropriate and consideration is given either to freeing a child for adoption or to an application for adoption which may be disputed, the child and adolescent psychiatrist should consider advising that, rather than terminating contact before adoption, every effort should be made to support it, if necessary in a neutral setting, while at the same time advising the parents about the needs and rights of the child to a permanent, secure home. The parents must be advised to seek legal advice and it will be up to them to demonstrate to the local authority and if necessary attempt to prove to the court that it is possible for them to offer the child a secure, satisfactory and permanent home by a defined date. If a court finds that this objective has not been achieved, contact should be reconsidered or terminated in the context of an adoption or freeing for adoption order.

A psychiatrist should be in a position to comment on the time scale for any rehabilitation effort in relation to the child's level of understanding and attachment needs. He or she could advise on factors relevant to a court decision that a parent was unreasonably withholding consent to freeing for adoption or adoption. These would be if a parent:

(a) had neglected or abused the child and had shown no evidence of change in attitude and behaviour
(b) was unable to offer the child a home and, with the child being in care:
    (i)   had made inadequate effort to cooperate with the local authority on a reasonable plan for rehabilitation
    (ii) had continued to neglect or abuse the child
    (iii) had failed to maintain contact
    (iv) had failed to attend for recommended psychiatric or other treatment for parent, child or family, or where treatment had been unsuccessful and
    (v) there seemed no reasonable prospect of the parent making a home for the child within a time-scale consonant with the child's developmental needs.

While feeling compassion for parents, who possibly through no fault of their own, have been unable to parent their children adequately, the child and adolescent psychiatrist must nevertheless keep firmly in mind an overriding duty to advise on the least detrimental solution for the child. This is likely to be, for children denied the prospect of a home with 'good-enough' natural parents, a home with permanent substitute parents.

In some cases an 'adoption with contact' arrangement can be made, usually for older children who wish to continue to have contact with parents who are unable to offer them a home, or with other key family members such as grandparents, and where the prospective adoptive parents are willing and able to allow this. This area can cause much heart-searching for the child and adolescent psychiatrist when natural justice seems to conflict with the child's needs. The judge will be the ultimate arbiter in this conflict and child and adolescent psychiatrists should make it clear that their expertise is not in civil rights but in child development and psychopathology. Child and adolescent psychiatrists are advised to remain on the alert for revision of the law concerning adoption (see also Chapter 13 on long-term substitute care).

Transracial and transcultural fostering and adoption

The literature on this subject has been reviewed by Zeitlin and colleagues and Harris-Hendriks & Figueroa (1995), who recommend, inter alia, that in assessments relevant to fostering or adoption, child and adolescent psychiatrists should consider the psychological effects of cultural and religious practice, social translocation, membership of a minority group, identity formation, self-esteem, the effects of social pressure and negative discrimination and, separately, the relevance to mental health of physical characteristics (including skin colour), race or culture of origin, attachment needs, and the social and cultural experiences of the child (Harris-Hendriks & Figueroa, 1995).

Psychiatric assessment, planning, placement, management and treatment of children should as far as possible be based on the results of research and empirical evidence rather than on political beliefs.

Where a child has had previous experience or knowledge of a particular culture, language or religion, he or she should be placed where possible in a family which will enable retention of such experience or knowledge as well as the acquisition of skills necessary for participating in the wider community of which he or she is a member.

When assessing a child and offering advice about placement, the child's self-perception, age and understanding should be taken into account.

Evidence suggests that transcultural adoption or foster placements in themselves should not lead to significant negative effects on the child. Other factors such as the stability of the placement, awareness of the child's needs by the substitute parents and their willingness to encourage open and frank discussion of the child's own cultural background are of greater importance. Adoptive and foster parents should be advised to help children develop a positive identity based on personal skills and attributes rather than solely on skin colour or identification with a minority group and to help them deal with negative discrimination.

Stability, quality and security of parenting, as well as speed of placement, should be given high priority in all cases and especially with young children. Consideration of attachment needs is essential and should take priority over other considerations such as race and culture.

Child and adolescent psychiatrists may find themselves having to argue that the needs of the child are more complex than can be solved merely by recruiting substitute parents with the same colour skin or religion, and that to accord one feature of the child overriding importance in matching that child to adoptive parents is to do violence to that complexity. It is essential to be familiar with the literature in this field (Gill & Jackson, 1984; Harris, 1985; Hersov, 1990; Tizard & Phoenix, 1990, 1993; James & Harris, 1994; Harris-Hendriks & Figueroa, 1995).

Long-term fostering, residence orders and adoption

When a child is the subject of a care order, child and adolescent psychiatrists may be involved in advising on the relative advantages for the child of these options (see Chapter 13). Residence orders are based on the fundamental principle that where the child lives should interfere as little as possible with relationships with parents and that contact with a wide range of important key relatives may be built into the plan for the child's future. There are obvious and well-documented disadvantages in long-term fostering (Bohman, 1981; Berridge & Cleaver, 1987; Aldgate, 1990), since parental responsibility for day-to-day care and for longer-term issues such as the child's health and education are shared uneasily between the state, represented by social workers, natural parents and foster carers. Where adoption is not an option, a residence order in favour of foster carers, with agreed contact between the child and the birth family or other key adults, may be a way of resolving some of these difficulties. (This would replace a care order.) Foster parents can be helped by continued financial support from a local authority combined with more emphasis on the permanency of the placement. Children can be represented in court by a guardian ad litem when decisions concerning these issues are being made. Adoption is the provision giving maximum security to a child unable to live with the family of origin.

Deportation orders

Sometimes a child is born in the UK to an illegal immigrant or to an applicant for refugee status and his or her civil and legal rights are impinged upon when a deportation order is made in respect of the parent or parents. Such cases should be heard urgently, in the highest tier of court, and it may be appropriate for a child and adolescent psychiatrist to assess the needs of the child concerned.

'Open' adoption and residence: a literature review

(*Note:* This section is relevant also to Chapter 7 on contact.)

During the 1990s, since the publication of *Patterns and Outcome in Child Placement* (Department of Health, 1991*b*), the courts have paid much closer attention to the issue of continuing contact, direct or indirect, with natural parents when agreeing long-term substitute care. The research findings described in this volume require close scrutiny before application to a specific case. The main message from recent follow-up studies is that children who are accommodated long-term benefit from *some form* of contact with their natural parents. However, as children are not randomly selected for adoption versus long-term foster care, and few adopted children have maintained *direct* contact with their parents, we still know little about the long-term outcome of open adoption. Most of the experience of open adoption stems from New Zealand (Rochel & Ryburn, 1988). This, together with studies monitoring legislation on access to birth records by adoptees (Mullender, 1991), suggests that, while face to face contact is not always desirable or practical, other forms of contact such as information, life-story work, letters and the preservation of links which permit contact to resume at a later date if the child or young adult wishes it are important (McCartt & Ohman Proch, 1993). A small study (Fratter *et al*, 1991) concluded that a child's need for contact does not necessarily conflict with the achievement of permanence and security in an alternative long-term home.

The common dilemma frequently faced by social workers and child and adolescent psychiatrists with very disturbed older children, or large sibling groups who cannot return to their natural parents, is the choice between closed adoption or open adoption or long-term fostering with continuation of direct contact. Attempts to seek adopters (Lambert *et al*, 1990) for such hard-to-place children may be more difficult if face to face contact is part of the plan, and delays in finding a permanent family often occur. The family of origin may in any case discontinue contact after adoption. We know that the risk of placement breakdown rises steeply with the age of children, longer periods in care and previous placement breakdown (Department of Health, 1991*b*), therefore a strategic decision needs to be made between permanent fostering arrangements and attempts to find adopters. Fratter (1991) *et al* suggests that permanent foster placements do not break down more often than adoptive placements when age is taken into account. This is at variance with the findings for young children (Aldgate, 1990; Department of Health, 1991*b*) that stability of placement and educational achievement are much greater for adoption than long-term foster care.

Since the introduction of the Children Act 1989, local authorities have tended to maintain high levels of contact between children and their natural parents before long-term decisions about placement are finalised. The findings of Rowe *et al* (1989) and Millham *et al* (1986, 1989) are still applicable now so that as in the past contact may lapse as a result of social work policies or omissions (such that sometimes even the completion of life histories has not been achieved). Outcomes of short- and long-term placements made prior to the Children Act 1989 suggested that children's well-being was enhanced by regular and frequent contact with parents (Department of Health, 1991*b*). This included the adoption of children with special needs (Fratter *et al*, 1991). What is unclear is whether these findings were influenced by qualities in both the carers and natural parents who may have struggled to maintain contact despite lack of active support from the local authority.

Other work (Department of Health, 1991*b*; Wedge & Mantle, 1991) suggests that the maintenance of direct contact between siblings in care, when whole sibling groups cannot be placed together, is of great importance. This is less likely to prove a hindrance to the recruitment of permanent carers or adopters than is the requirement of continued direct contact with parents. Practitioners will need to consider the individual needs of older disturbed or developmentally delayed children and the likelihood of finding a permanent family for a large sibling group within a reasonable time frame. One way of ensuring more rapid placement is to encourage social workers to advertise children as a sibling group but also encouraging applicants to apply for part of the group providing they are committed to maintaining contact.

Summary

Planning for the long term is essential whenever a child may be or is received into care by a local authority. The plan should include a programme for maintaining the child in his or her home or for attempted rehabilitation, a time-scale, and provision for what happens if the plan fails. A child, or foster carers, should not be allowed to drift from 'short-term' to longer-term care without planning since the effect on all parties can be damaging in the extreme. It may be a psychiatrist's responsibility to spell out clearly the consequences when such bad practices are found and to suggest ways of ending them. It is now possible to state that it is preferable for a child to be adopted than to stay in long-term unplanned care or, except for clearly defined, well-argued reasons, to be in an institution. Child and adolescent psychiatrists should be familiar with the literature supporting these views (Tizard, 1987; Hersov, 1994; Wolkind, 1994).

Criteria for assessing placement programmes

(a) Have parents cooperated fully with the programme? Is the programme realistic?
(b) Has there been any improvement or deterioration in the child's and family's functioning? This is assessed by:
    (i) psychological and psychiatric assessments of child and family
    (ii) school, nursery and social work reports, records of height and weight and paediatric examination, as appropriate.
(c) Has the programme kept roughly to time; if not, have the reasons for delay been acceptable?
(d) Are long-term objectives clear-cut, achievable and well monitored?

Check-list

If consulted in a dispute about where a child should live, with whom the child can have contact, or whether he or she should be freed for adoption, or in a disputed adoption hearing, consider the following.

(a) Has an adequate plan for attempted rehabilitation been devised and vigorously pursued by the local authority?
(b) If not, advise on:
    (i) feasibility
    (ii) time-scale in relation to developmental stage of the child

  (iii) the child's attachment needs
  (iv) existing relationships
   (v) treatment needs of all parties.
(c) If a plan has been tried and has failed, consider the child's needs for contact while 'freeing' procedures are initiated, and how your recommendation may be implemented.
(d) Factors which a court would consider relevant in deciding whether a parent was or was not unreasonably withholding consent to the adoption of a child in care would be if a parent had:
    (i) failed to cooperate with attempted rehabilitation plan
   (ii) failed to maintain contact
  (iii) continued to neglect or abuse the child
   (iv) failed to attend for recommended treatment
    (v) not benefited from treatment within a reasonable time
   (vi) not been able to make a home for the child within a reasonable time
  (vii) based objections to the adoption solely on racial, religious or other restrictive considerations, and had failed to consider the best interests of the child in the long term
 (viii) been considered to be unable to benefit from treatments available which might modify his or her 'dangerousness' (in relation to placing a child at risk of 'significant harm').

10 Compensation claims

Compensation may be claimed where it is thought that a personal injury secondary to an event involving crime or negligence on the part of another (the defendant) has caused damage to a child (the plaintiff). In this context, damage refers to both financial loss and significant physical or psychological harm, loss of capacity, or increased risk of future psychiatric disorder. It is also possible to claim for loss of a parent through death or injury. A named person or institution can be held responsible and sued for damages. Negligence requires there to be a 'duty of care' owed to the plaintiff by the defendant who should have foreseen the possibility of the plaintiff's injury, taking the plaintiff as he finds him without allowance for idiosyncratic vulnerability (an 'eggshell personality'). It then needs to be shown that negligence is causally related to the damage. The 'quantum' of damages is composed of direct financial loss and non-financial losses such as suffering or the possible future cost of treatment. The child and adolescent psychiatrist offers expert opinion on the description of the damage, its causal relation to the event, the prognosis and, often, on any adverse impact upon future social adjustment including adult earnings. Psychiatric opinion can also assist the court or the two sides in the estimation of the cost of financial and non-financial loss and the likelihood of future psychiatric treatment.

Individual children can sue the defendant, through a 'next friend' (usually a parent). On occasion (as in a shipping or train accident) there may be an action on behalf of a number of children. If a child has been the victim of a crime, he or she can apply to the Criminal Injuries Compensation Authority for compensation. Although adults need to make a claim within three years of a traumatic criminal event, children have an extended time in which to do so. They may claim compensation following an event occurring at any time in their childhood so long as their claim is made within three years after reaching the age of 18.

As far as claims following criminal acts are concerned, the Official Solicitor to the Supreme Court regularly acts on behalf of children who make a claim but relatives, social workers, police and guardians ad litem may initiate a claim and may indeed be negligent if they do not consider this option (Criminal Injuries Compensation Board (now Authority), 1989). Claims may be made whether or not there has been a criminal trial or despite the outcome of a trial. The claim is based on having suffered a criminal injury, not on the attribution of responsibility for the cause of that injury.

The event leading to a claim may have involved actual or suspected physical injury to the child which might be associated with subsequent loss of psychological function or psychiatric disorder. Instances include head injury, cerebral hypoxia during medical procedures, physical injury with adverse cosmetic consequences, or putative brain injury suffered during childbirth. Alternatively what is in question is whether a manifestly unpleasant and apparently traumatic experience has given rise to psychological consequences which go beyond understandable distress. The latter can include post-traumatic stress disorder (PTSD) or phobic reactions.

When psychological damage accompanies physical damage, the cost of one is added to the other. If a traumatic experience results solely in psychological damage in the form of an emotional reaction this needs to extend beyond ordinary pain and suffering ('normal mere emotions') and be related to the direct experience of a traumatic event in order to qualify as 'nervous shock'. The latter is an old but still current concept, now often taken as roughly equivalent to PTSD which is not quite correct; it applies to any psychiatric diagnosis which follows from direct experience of (close proximity to) a traumatic incident.

The request for a report

Requests for psychiatric reports are nearly always made to an independent psychiatrist by a private solicitor who will have details of the event relevant to litigation. The solicitor may represent litigant or defendant. This is the preferred mode of referral since it places the psychiatrist in a single role, grants possession of the facts of the case and clarifies payment of fees. Occasionally a psychiatrist who is already involved clinically with the child is approached for a report by a solicitor or parent. More insidiously, a referral, ostensibly for treatment, is sought by parents though the issue of a report is raised subsequently and it becomes clear that it was the covert reason for referral.

It may be wise to decline to write a report when clinically involved as the nature of the contract between psychiatrist, child and parents is different in the two instances. Assessment for a report may require the psychiatrist to question or disqualify the views and even the evidence of the child or parents in a manner which would run counter to the formation or maintenance of a treatment alliance. Furthermore, it specifically does not provide the child and parents with confidentiality and the relationship is no longer one of doctor and patient. There is also the risk that once the claim is settled the family will break off treatment prematurely.

With this in mind, it may well be preferable for an expert report on a child who is already a patient of one psychiatrist to be prepared by another psychiatrist and the reasons for this explained. Clearly this reservation does not apply to reports in which the psychiatrist is a witness to fact and not required to express an expert opinion.

The request process and relationship with the solicitor differs from proceedings brought under the Children Act 1989. The legal process is openly adversarial when personal injury litigation is concerned and there are rules and timetables for the exchange of reports. Psychiatric and other expert reports may not eventually be disclosed to the other side and it is incorrect for an expert witness on one side to approach a witness for the other. It may be necessary eventually to omit a mention of certain reports in any list of sources of information since the solicitor may not wish to disclose these to the other side. The final report should not be sent to anyone, including the child's general practitioner, without the permission of the solicitor, although one should write to a general practitioner, with the parents' agreement, if urgent and treatable clinical conditions are uncovered by psychiatric assessment.

An initial approach for a report may be tentative, asking in principle whether you would have the appropriate expertise and be able to prepare a report. If only minimal details of the case are available it is obviously wise to be a little cautious, ask for further information, clarification of what legal questions require an answer, provide an estimate of your fee, based on a stated hourly rate, and say when you could provide the report. Legal aid clearance for your fees will often be required if you are reporting on a litigant and it is necessary to wait for this to be granted. The solicitor who negotiates it will often take a month or more before giving the go-ahead. The family will need a couple of weeks' notice of an appointment so that a tentative diary booking of an appointment time can be made for about six weeks ahead. It is, incidentally, not uncommon for families not to attend appointments or to cancel at the last minute.

Personal injury ('PI') litigation is often a drawn-out process, not usually to the psychological benefit of the child. With this in mind a comprehensive assessment and full written report is essential as it may not be used until a year or more later. Early in the litigation process it may not be possible for the solicitor to indicate a date for the court hearing. In practice, less than 5% of child personal injury litigation goes to court and a settlement on the steps of the court is not unknown. If a court date is available, organise your diary accordingly, advise the solicitor of your charge for attending and charge for any cancellation of a requirement to attend. This can be on a sliding scale: one month, one week and one day before, according to the inconvenience or loss of earning that you would experience. Stating terms for this (and charges for appointments not kept) before the request is accepted saves difficulties later.

A definitive request should state what points need to be addressed and will usually be accompanied by some documentation of the event in question. There may be other information available and this can be made available to you. Consider general practice and school records in nearly every case. There may also be reports from medical and other experts. A telephone discussion with the solicitor can help here. Your opinion will be much stronger if you can demonstrate independent corroboration or disconfirmation of the child and family's account, or there may be factors prior to the event in question which need consideration.

The assessment process

It is clearly important to establish:

    (a) what the child was like before the event
    (b) what happened during the event
    (c) what the child has been like subsequently and whether a psychiatric disorder is present
    (d) whether there is a causal link between the event and subsequent or present state
    (e) the grounds for estimating prognosis.

Both written records and clinical interviews with parent(s) and child will provide information. As far as the clinical interview is concerned, it is sensible to see parents and child together initially to explain the purpose of the interview and how the rules of confidentiality differ from the ordinary process of seeing a doctor. It is subsequently often appropriate to see parents separately and the child individually, testing for consistency between separate accounts. In practice, faking is very unusual but it is wise to demonstrate a cautious approach.

Which aspect to start with needs a little thought. The circumstances of the event may be asked about first in order to establish exactly with child and parents what the report is about. Nevertheless, some children and parents will find this distressing and this can disrupt interviewing. It is sensible to ask whether the interviewee would like to talk about the event and respect a wish not to. There will nearly always be a written account of the event available.

With this in mind, a developmental history up to the time of the event may be selected as the first area of enquiry. This can provide a baseline against which the impact of the event can be assessed. Multiple sources of information help. School and general practice records can usually be obtained through the solicitor.

The child's condition shortly after the event may be particularly important; it can indicate the emotional or physical impact of the event and forms a subsidiary baseline against which subsequent progress can be assessed. This is helpful in considering prognosis. If contemporaneous hospital records exist they should be requested and examined closely.

Parents may unwittingly bias their account of their child's reaction. In other than head injury cases (where the need for adequate funds to guarantee the child's future welfare is obvious), it is very unusual for a desire for money to be a stated motive in litigation. More commonly, parents want the defendant to apologise or acknowledge their negligence. They often have a preconceived idea that the event has caused their child's current difficulty and their presentation of information can be coloured by this. On the other hand, some parents who have been involved in traumatic experiences will minimise the impact upon the child, probably in an effort to reassure themselves that the child is emotionally unharmed. With this in mind, seeking independent documentation of changes in the child is extremely important.

Clearly the child's current capacities, behaviour and mental state must be examined. A mental state examination is crucial. The content of memories, dreams or preoccupations will be important in establishing a link with traumatic experiences. Assessment of such elements as memory, cognitive capacity and concentration will be a central part of examining a child with a past head injury. Full exploration of aspects such as fearful avoidance behaviour or social disinhibition respectively will need an account (with specific examples) from a parent. Correlation between observed behaviour and stated emotion need examining. For instance a child may deny the adverse impact of a cosmetically challenging scar while going to some lengths to conceal it by hair or clothing during the interview. Manifest arousal indicated by observed changes in respiration, pulse rate in the neck, lip dryness or pupil size while recalling a traumatic event may be at variance with a 'brave' child who minimises their own upset.

Listening to the phrases used by the child in describing their own experiences may reveal a stereotyped nature or unusually adult phraseology suggesting 'priming' by parents, though this is very unusual to encounter. Some estimate of the child's suggestibility should be made by observing how easily he or she can be led by questioning. Competence as a witness may be assessed by discussion of recent, non-traumatic life events.

Drawings, play or asking the child to re-enact the event may provide cogent evidence of suffering underestimated by parents and teachers, as may careful history-taking relevant to the concept of post-traumatic stress (see Chapter 8).

Tracking changes in emotional reactions or behaviour by obtaining precise dates or ages will allow assessment as to whether the event made a material contribution to present distress or disability. The severity of emotional or behavioural change requires quantification as the question as to whether these are normal reactions or go beyond 'ordinary pain and suffering'.

It may be necessary to ask for neuropsychological assessment, imaging studies or other tests. The cost of these is likely to be substantial and not be contained within your estimated fee. Accordingly, the need for these should be discussed with the solicitor before commissioning them.

Writing the report

The introduction should follow the principles set out in Chapter 3, setting out the grounds for your opinion being seen as expert, explaining the purpose of the report, and the sources of information. Some care is needed with the latter as the solicitor may not eventually wish to disclose these to the other side. Rather than have to alter the pagination of your report it may be easier to refer to a separate list included as an appendix which can be amended easily if subsequently necessary.

There is something to be said for setting out the report in sections under headings, for example: introduction; the child before the event; the event itself; the child immediately after the event; the child now; conclusion as to causation; prognosis.

This is not rigid. For instance there may also be specific legal questions which the solicitor has asked to be addressed. In some cases it may be better to state your conclusions at the end of each section, building your argument accordingly. Clearly the above structure would not apply to a case in which an opinion on an expert report from the other side is all that is requested.

Careful distinction between information and opinion is obviously necessary. It is generally agreed that a reasoned opinion, constructed in stages with respect to the findings and their interpretation is preferable to an intuitive response based on so many years of experience. With this in mind, phrases such as "I feel..." might be better omitted.

If a psychiatric disorder is present, reference to the evidence for it is best tied to ICD–10 (World Health Organization, 1992) (especially the research edition which contains itemised operational definitions) or DSM–IV (American Psychiatric Association, 1994) and this made explicit, referring your findings to the chosen criteria. For nervous shock to be demonstrated, a psychiatric diagnosis is essential. There are difficulties with anxiety conditions which fall short of PTSD but nevertheless include fearful avoidance of circumstance reminiscent of the event, sleep disturbances and an emergent insecurity of attachment. Quite often these last for longer than the six-month period within which adjustment disorder is diagnosable and current classification schemes cannot easily accommodate them without recourse to not otherwise stated categories.

The question as to how current psychiatric disorder might be related to the event in question may be interpreted differently according to legal and psychiatric principles. For instance, a child who was asleep during a horrific road traffic accident may be psychologically affected because his mother is suffering from PTSD. His disorder clearly relates ultimately to the event but does not stem directly from his experience of it and will not be nervous shock.

The current level of disability, suffering or restriction of activities needs to be stated explicitly.

If psychiatric treatment is required but not readily available through the NHS, then the costs of private treatment should be spelled out by, for instance, indicating the number of sessions likely to be needed and the rate per session.

Lawyers sometimes ask for precise quantification of future risk. Psychiatrists are not used to this and some recourse to phrases such as "it is more likely than not..." may be wiser than venturing a spuriously accurate percentage. If it not clear what the prognosis will be, suggest alternative measures such as an interim settlement or establishing a contingency fund. It may be important to press for an early settlement on clinical grounds.

If necessary at any point in the report, quote references to support any conclusion, as in a piece of academic writing. It is obviously not necessary to justify every remark. It is courteous to provide the solicitor with a reprint or photocopy of the article cited.

Remember that the parents will see what you have written. If you have observations about their reliability or their mental states it may be better to telephone the solicitor or write a separate letter, asking that it be treated in confidence.

Subsequent events

After submitting the report there may be a long period of silence. There may then come a request to change certain parts of the report once the parents or counsel have seen it. Clearly these requests need to be taken on their merits. A factual error which can be shown to be just that should be changed but an amendment to opinion might be rightly resisted. Requests to delete references to reports from other experts which will not be disclosed are perfectly reasonable, given the legal rules governing litigation procedure.

The other side may solicit their own expert opinions and you may be asked to comment on these. The points about which you disagree are less important than identifying weaknesses in the arguments used in their reports as this will provide ammunition for the lawyers on the side which engaged you.

At some point there may be a conference in chambers with a barrister. Reading one's own report beforehand is the minimum preparation as matters will often be conducted in a brisk manner, time being chargeable. Take your own notes as it may be some time before the agreed strategy comes to court – if it ever does. It is appropriate to charge for your own time when attending such a conference.

Litigation proceeds slowly and it may be necessary for you to review your report a year or two later at the invitation of the solicitor, re-interviewing the child as appropriate and submitting a supplementary report.

Check-list

(a) Is psychopathology present beyond a proportionate response? What is its nature and severity?
(b) Does it conform to a recognised diagnosis in ICD–10 or DSM–IV?

(c) Was it present before the event in question?
(d) What factors contribute to its aetiology? Did the event contribute materially to its causation?
(e) What, if anything, contributes to its maintenance?
(f) What restrictions does it impose upon the child now and in the future?
(g) Are there financial constraints such as relative loss of earnings?
(h) Is it amenable to treatment and if so, what kind and how extensive?
(i) Is this readily available on the NHS or how much will it cost?
(j) What is the likely prognosis, with and without treatment?
(k) Are any further investigations or assessments required?

11 Education

Each local education authority (LEA) interprets education law to suit local conditions, so it may be advisable to contact a principal education psychologist or special schools placement officer of the relevant LEA when it is necessary to clarify details of local practice. All work with individual children and their families must be undertaken according to the principles outlined in Chapter 5.

Non-attendance

Since the Education Act (England and Wales) 1870 became law, education has been compulsory. This was regarded as a major social reform primarily intended to promote literacy, obedience and punctuality.

The Education Act 1996 requires children to "receive education according to their age, aptitude and ability", LEAs to provide such education, and parents to ensure that their children are educated. The law now requires children to receive education from the beginning of the term after their fifth birthday, until a date around their 16th birthday. If the birthday falls between 1 September and 31 January the child may not leave until the end of the Easter term. If the birthday falls between 1 February and 31 August the child may leave at the summer half-term. Many LEAs offer school commencement before the age of five and all children reaching the appropriate education standards or with special needs are entitled to education beyond the age of 16. Offences are referred to as 'non-attendance' but this could be restated as 'failure to receive education' or 'failure to ensure that a child receives education'. If a child is not on a school roll a prosecution for non-attendance cannot be brought.

Parents may if they wish provide education other than through the state system of schools. All schools, including those privately run, are open to inspection, now undertaken on behalf of the

Government by a regulatory agency, the Office for Standards in Education (OFSTED). If the child is educated at home, the local authority has a duty to monitor and satisfy itself that the child is receiving an education appropriate to his or her needs. The school year runs from September to August and comprises 200 school days arranged into three terms. Statutory school registers are maintained and regularly reviewed by the LEA. Education welfare officers have a duty to investigate if children are not attending school and to take appropriate action.

Children may of course miss school for a number of legitimate reasons such as illness, family crises and for holidays agreed between parents and the headteacher (within guidelines provided by the LEA). Unacceptable non-attendance occurs for a variety of reasons and provides, with parental consent, an appropriate field for liaison between education welfare officers, education psychologists, children's lawyers and child and family psychiatric services. Sometimes a court will request a psychiatric report when a child or parent is before it for non-attendance.

Absence from school

School refusal

Persistent absence from school may be linked with emotional disorder. Children in this category are described as suffering from 'school refusal'. Characteristically they stay at home when they should be at school. Symptoms of anxiety and depression occur and may be mistaken for those of physical illness. Emotional upset at the prospect of having to attend school is apparent.

Children who suffer from school refusal are usually dealt with by educational, medical or psychological agencies according to local referral practices and the particular features of the case. Thus school refusal masquerading as physical illness may lead to extensive investigations by family doctors and paediatricians before the true nature of the condition is realised. Child and adolescent psychiatrists commonly treat school refusal on an out-patient basis and early return to school generally is recommended. Admission to hospital day units or in-patient units sometimes may be considered necessary.

When the nature of the condition is understood and parents cooperate in the process of treatment the education authorities do not unnecessarily take legal action. However, children and adolescents who refuse school may be taken before the juvenile court and, if the case is proven, an education supervision order may be made (Children Act 1989). It is no longer possible to make a care order solely on the grounds of non-attendance at school.

Parents of these children may also be prosecuted in the magistrates' court. This can happen when the true nature of the problem is not appreciated by the education authority or when parents do not recognise the need for, or cooperate with, appropriate treatment. Sometimes parents blame the school for their child's problem and actively condone absence. They may demand home tuition or placement at a particular school when neither of those alternatives is in the best interest of the child. Sometimes, in these circumstances, a child and adolescent psychiatrist is asked to submit a court report or give evidence during the court proceedings to explain the nature of school refusal to the magistrates and describe the treatment recommended. Sometimes treatment may be offered more effectively when the child is subject to a supervision order (see Berg & Nursten, 1996).

Truancy

Truancy, failure to go to school as legally required, is often associated with conduct disorder. Such children steal, tell lies, fight excessively, show destructiveness and have difficulty in forming normal relationships with their peers. Educational backwardness and disruptiveness in school often are associated. Truants attempt to conceal from their families the fact that they are not at school. Care orders may be made only when factors additional to non-attendance are significant.

Problems of this kind are less susceptible to a therapeutic approach but may improve under pressure from the school authorities and courts or changes in educational provision and management. Harris (1987), Grenville (1988) and Berg & Nursten (1996) review the legal, ethical and research issues relevant to the use of repeated adjournments in cases of persistent truancy. From time to time child and adolescent psychiatrists are asked to provide reports for the juvenile court on a child who is truanting. Suggestions concerning special educational placements and support required by the family can be included in the report, which should contain an opinion as to the presence or absence of conduct disorder and other psychiatric disorders in the child.

School withdrawal or condoned absence

Sometimes failure to attend school appears to be due to deliberate encouragement, by irresponsible or over-protective parents, for the child to remain away from school. Repeated inadequate explanations may be offered. No evidence may emerge of either neurotic disorder or conduct disorder affecting the child. The families are usually rather deprived materially, and disorganised. When not at school children may be employed with household tasks such as caring for younger brothers and sisters. Highly mobile families may fail to enrol their children at school and others avoid prosecution by changes of residence.

Mixed pictures

Children involved in court proceedings because of failure to attend school do not always fit neatly into categories, or there may be insufficient information for classification. It is by no means uncommon for children to show mixed pictures with, for example, antisocial behaviour and truancy being prominent at one time and evidence of emotional disorder and school refusal or masquerade syndrome taking precedence at another. Some degree of parental condoning of absence may be found in truancy, as in school refusal. Psychiatric reports should indicate which features are clearly evident and which are not and weigh up the balance of probabilities regarding the presented attendance problem. Recommendations for management while the child either remains at home or is received into care will be of help to the magistrates.

Suspension and exclusion from school

The head of a school has the power to exclude, for short and fixed periods, a pupil who has behaved unacceptably: the pupil may be prevented temporarily from attending school. A child may only be excluded for indefinite periods or permanently by authority of the school governors, a statutory body for each school, with responsibilities in law for the governance of that school and interested in the whole process of education. They may order the removal of a child's name from the school roll, the decision being ratified where relevant by the education officer of the local authority concerned. Such decisions are subject to appeal by parents or guardians and may be over-ruled.

The consequences of such a decision are monitored by education welfare officers, often in consultation with educational psychologists who in turn, with the consent of parents, may consult a child and adolescent psychiatric service. This process may lead to informal problem solving or the provisions of the Education Act 1996 may be invoked on behalf of the child and family.

A child psychiatric service may advise the family, the school and the court about available and appropriate therapeutic interventions and, in consultation with relevant colleagues within the education department, may consider the need for additional educational provision. An opinion may be offered regarding relationships within the family and the degree to which parents and child may cooperate with plans for the child's education.

It will be appropriate, often, to give an opinion that the child concerned is not suffering from any psychiatric illness such as to prevent attendance at school.

Special educational needs

The Education Act 1981 (England and Wales) was implemented in April 1983. It did away with the former 10 special educational categories (such as 'maladjusted') of pupils with special needs. Instead, it requires all professionals dealing with the child to write advice concerning these needs. The child's parents have the right to see this advice and to make representations concerning their child. The resultant 'statement of special educational needs' has added a new transitive verb, 'to statement', to the English language. This Statement is the collation of all advice received and must specify the appropriate school or other provision to meet the identified needs of the child. Parents may appeal, first to the local authority's education officer, then to the courts and finally to the Department for Education and Employment, if they disagree with a local authority's decision as 'statemented' (Department of Health and Social Security, 1983a). If the child is not the subject of a statement under the Education Act 1996 the parent may apply for an assessment under the Act and the authority shall comply unless it considers the request unreasonable (section 9).

Child and adolescent psychiatric services may contribute to such assessments, including the child and family in all stages of the assessment procedure. Written recommendations are available to the parents as well as to other professionals concerned in planning on behalf of the child. Psychiatrists may wish also to comment on delays in implementing decisions or on the availability of resources.

The Education Reform Act (England and Wales) 1988 and subsequent legislation created financial and structural changes in the provision of education. In particular, local education authorities hold smaller budgets, with management of much day-to-day educational provision being devolved to schools and their governors. Special education provision may be more erratic, less in quantity and more variable between educational authorities than hitherto. Multi-disciplinary cooperation, so necessary to the effective provision of health and educational services to children in need, will require the development and maintenance of new communication systems between service providers.

The Education Act (England and Wales) 1996 contains a Code of Practice on Special Educational Needs and a right of appeal against refusal by an education authority to assess a child or to issue a statement or on the content of a statement. Children have the right to special education according to their needs until they reach their 19th birthday.

Any child who does not make effective use of the available education system may require help based on a complex and expanding field of knowledge comprising education, law, psychology, social work, paediatrics and psychiatry. The resource implications are substantial (Bennathan, 1992).

Check-list

(a) The psychiatrist should achieve a working relationship with the appropriate education psychology service and special schools placement officers.

(b) Child and adolescent psychiatrists should be familiar with local educational practices arising from application of the Code of Practice for Special Educational Needs required to be considered under the Education Act 1996.

(c) Issues of confidentiality should be considered as outlined in Chapter 5.

(d) When working on 'special needs' assessments of children (Department of Health and Social Security, 1983*a*) the psychiatrist should obtain consent from, and write statements of need in a form acceptable to the parents or guardians concerned.

(e) When asked for a court report concerning non-attendance the psychiatrist should use the check-list in Chapter 3.

12 Juvenile justice

The specialised form of magistrates' court dealing primarily with criminal proceedings relating to children and young people has been renamed the Youth Court and now brings 17-year-olds within its jurisdiction, thus bringing England and Wales into line with other European countries (Criminal Justice Act 1991 (England & Wales)).

The Youth Court consists of two or three magistrates (including one man and one woman) drawn from a special panel of lay justices from the local community. They are appointed by the Crown on the advice of the Lord Chancellor and although not legally qualified receive special training. They sit with a legally qualified clerk who advises them on points of law. Chapter 3 advises about court appearances.

It is usual for a psychiatric report to be requested after a 'finding of guilt' (not conviction) in order to help the magistrates decide an 'order on finding of guilt' (not sentence). In such cases the request is made on behalf of the Bench either by a social worker or by a probation officer.

Consent in such cases from children and parents is not necessary. In all other circumstances the psychiatrist should seek appropriate consent and also find out whether what is being requested is an expert or professional opinion (see Chapter 1). It is more usual for a psychiatrist to be asked for an expert opinion particularly in relation to bizarre, unusual or dangerous offences. Psychiatrists specialising in this branch of forensic psychiatry should be alert to prospective legislation concerning crime and disorder.

Delinquency

(a) A young person found guilty of a crime is a juvenile delinquent. Delinquency is a socio-legal, not a psychiatric, category. The standard definition of a juvenile delinquent is a young person between the age of 10 and 17 years who has been prosecuted and found guilty of an offence that would be classified as a crime if committed by an adult. Such offences lead to a criminal conviction record in the central files at Scotland Yard.

(b) Research findings are consistent in showing that the majority of young people (particularly boys) have committed 'delinquent' acts at some time (West & Farrington, 1973; West, 1982). West (1982) showed that the vast majority of offences were crimes of dishonesty involving theft, driving away vehicles without the owner's consent, breaking into premises with intent to steal, and destructive vandalism, technically 'criminal damage'. Collectively these account for over 90% of recorded juvenile offences. Crimes of personal violence and drug and sex offences constitute a very small proportion of juvenile offences, although these become relatively more common over the age of 17 years. West also showed that the majority of offences, especially those committed by juveniles, were small scale and relatively trivial, more of a nuisance than a serious threat; also that most of the offence histories seemed to reflect petty, disorganised, impulsive and generally unprofitable crimes. Many of these boys appear only in court once however and only a small proportion show a persistent path of delinquency.

The report

The report should be laid out as described in Chapter 3. It is important for psychiatrists to realise that a report may be read out in its entirety in court. They should consider the impact this could have on an adolescent and his or her family if the report has not been discussed with them in advance. It should be written in clear, accurate, even sympathetic language that does not alienate the adolescent and the family from the helping professions. An adolescent should not learn for the first time that he or she, or another family member, is suffering from a serious illness such as carcinoma or schizophrenia, or is illegitimate or adopted. This may be avoided by marking a paragraph 'confidential' and requesting that it be not read out in court.

When making a medical recommendation it is desirable to assess whether or not the adolescent is motivated to accept treatment and whether or not treatment can be offered. There is little point in recommending treatment for glue-sniffing if the adolescent has no motivation to change, nor in recommending analytically-orientated psychotherapy if suitable resources are not available. Support for recommendations such as care orders to the local authority who must agree to become a party to the proceedings or supervision by the probation service first must be discussed with the relevant social services or probation department. This contact can often be used constructively to share information and guidance about future management. A report should not recommend a particular disposal but should provide psychiatric guidance as to which might be helpful or unhelpful. Psychiatrists should be aware of this range and the way their reports might lead the magistrates to select a particular disposal. In particular, it is not the task of a doctor to recommend a custodial sentence.

Range of disposals

The Criminal Justice and Public Order Act 1994 (England and Wales) has introduced three major changes in sentencing. The Secure Training Order is a six-month to two-year sentence for 12–14-year-olds available to the Youth and Crown Courts, with the custodial sentence being served in Home Office (not child care) establishments. The maximum sentence of detention in a Young Offenders Institution has been increased (see below). Section 53 detention can be used for all young people from 10 years old upwards, with a widening of the range of relevant offences. A particular addition is the offence of indecent assault on a woman.

When a custodial sentence for a juvenile is being considered certain reports must be prepared before sentencing. The Criminal Justice Act 1991 renames Social Enquiry Reports as Pre-Sentence Reports, which should indicate a range of options, not definite recommendations to the court. The Act also states that the court shall obtain and consider a medical report before sentencing if the offender appears to be mentally disordered. Approval under Section 12(2) of the Mental Health Act 1983 is a necessary requisite for this work.

Caution

This is imposed by police, not by a court, but if the youngster offends again and appears in court, the court will be told of the previous caution.

Absolute discharge

This implies no guilt or punishment. As it is not the task of psychiatrists to prove or disprove guilt, this should never be recommended.

Conditional discharge

If a first non-serious or series of minor offences over a brief period has been committed and the child has 'learnt his lesson', then conditional discharge can be recommended. This can also be linked to an offer of treatment.

Adjournment *sine die*

The case is proven, but the court adjourns disposal to assess the response to some intervention, such as testing of school attendance, change in family structure, work experience, etc. This may be used in care proceedings, but is rarely used in criminal proceedings and in these cases the court is more likely to defer sentence or to adjourn to a fixed date.

Fines

The parent, not defendant, must pay fines, unless the court decides that this is unreasonable. As such, it is probably ineffective, for although it implies parental responsibility, usually it causes no inconvenience to the child. Parents must be allowed to express their views in court on this.

Bind-over child/parents to keep the peace

This can be imposed whether or not there is a finding of guilt, with or without financial penalty, but there may be a fine if the order is breached.

Compensation order

This can now be recommended as the sole sentence. As with fines, parents must be allowed to express their views in court.

Deprivation order

This is a punishment in which the child can be deprived of keys or tools used in the course of an offence.

Deferment of sentence

This is a more stringent response than is commonly recognised. After a defined period, the defendant is sentenced with due reference to his or her behaviour during that period.

Attendance centre

This requires deprivation of liberty on Saturdays for up to 24 hours, in two- to three-hour blocks. Centres are run by police and a breach of the order leads to automatic return to court. This is for boys only.

Care order, supervision order or probation order

Under the terms of the Children Act 1989, a care order may no longer be imposed as a sentence in criminal proceedings. However, the fact that a child has committed an offence may indicate that he or she is suffering, or is likely to suffer, significant harm, so that a local authority may apply for a care or supervision order in respect of that child. Supervision orders may still be made in criminal proceedings. The purpose of such orders is to give primary consideration to the need to safeguard and promote the welfare of the child. The protection of the public is a secondary consideration.

A care order can be made when a previously made supervision order in criminal proceedings has been deemed to provide the child with insufficient care and control.

These orders were originally introduced in the Children and Young Persons Act 1969 as a means of dealing with juvenile offenders through an intermediate treatment programme. Now they can be linked to a number of disposals (see below). The statutory responsibility lies with the local social services to "advise, assist and befriend". However, the supervisor has powers to give direction to the supervisee and to return him or her to court if the terms of the order are breached. A supervision order lasts for a maximum of three years, and cannot be extended beyond the age of 18 years.

Supervision order with additional requirements

Supervised activity requirement/retraining requirement

Magistrates can make this recommendation directly and social services have to accept it. The discretionary powers of social services in large part have been removed with regard to intermediate treatment orders since the enactment of the Criminal Justice Act 1982, although social workers can still recommend them.

Night restriction order

This imposes a curfew on a child to his or her home, ordered by magistrates, between 18.00 and 06.00 for a total of 10 hours within this period. It is rarely used because of the difficulty of enforcement.

Residence requirement

A child already subject to a supervision order, but living at home, who has committed a serious offence, can be directed by the court to be removed from home and placed elsewhere for up to six months.

'Refrain from' requirement

This is an extra condition forbidding attendance at certain places, for example football matches, amusement arcades, etc.

Parental requirements

Supervision orders may impose requirements on those with parental responsibility for the child, and on other people with whom the child is living.

Community service order

This is used for adolescents over 16 years old who are required to do 40–120 hours unpaid, socially useful work, supervised by the probation service, which must make an assessment before a recommendation is made. This is a serious alternative to detention in a young offender institution. Youths are called back to court if they do not comply within two weeks of beginning their contract.

Detention in young offender institutions

This replaced borstal and detention centre orders and youth custody sentences and from 1983 gave increased powers to magistrates (Criminal Justice Act 1982). They are for boys and girls from 15–17 years. The Criminal Justice and Public Order Act 1994 has increased the maximum sentence from 12 months to two years.

Committal to crown court following deferment of sentence

A youth who has previously received a deferred sentence, yet repeats offences, can now be sent to crown court for disposal.

Guardianship order

Where the child in need of psychiatric treatment is an out-patient, rights and duties are vested in the guardian (e.g. local authority) to ensure that such treatment is carried out. Both this and hospital orders require the evidence of two registered medical practitioners.

The same considerations apply as in the application of the Mental Health Act 1983 to adult offenders.

Psychiatric treatment

If treatment is recommended it is open to the magistrates to link this with another disposal. It could be linked to a supervision order under the Children Act 1989 for out-patient or in-patient treatment. The latter would apply to a mentally ill child and a particular hospital should be specified (see also Chapter 13).

Many delinquents have learning difficulties or specific developmental delay. The psychiatrist does not make any direct recommendations about the young person's schooling, but should strongly recommend that an educational assessment be arranged.

13   Children and the law

Each section of this chapter refers substantially to legislation in England and Wales. Principles for practice are relevant to other jurisdictions: it is essential that practitioners are familiar with the law within the jurisdiction in which they work. Harris-Hendriks (1993), Grounds (1995) and Cope (1995 a,b) contain accounts of the law in Scotland, Northern Ireland and Eire. Relevant references are included in the supplementary reading list.

Section I
Legal minors and consent to treatment (England and Wales)

Child and adolescent psychiatrists must consider the legal minors they work with in three capacities: informal patients, detained patients and mentally abnormal offenders. A new code of practice awaits publication.

Informal patients

It should be noted that the terms 'child', 'adolescent' and 'young person' are not used in the current mental health legislation. The term 'patient' is used throughout without distinction of age except in two specific instances.

(a) The Mental Health Act 1983 (England and Wales) section 10 states:

> 1. Nothing in this Act should be construed as preventing a patient who requires treatment for a mental disorder from being admitted to any hospital or mental nursing home in pursuance of arrangements made in that behalf and without any application, order or direction, rendering them liable to be detained under this Act or from remaining in any hospital or mental nursing home in pursuance of

such arrangements after he has ceased to be liable to be so detained.
2. In the case of a minor who has attained the age of sixteen years
and is capable of expressing his own wishes, any such arrangements
as are made in subsection 1 (above) will be made, carried out and
determined notwithstanding any right of custody or control vested
in law by his parent or guardian.

(b) This is congruent with the Family Law Reform Act (England and
Wales) 1969, section 8, which states that the consent of a minor, who
has attained the age of 16, to medical or dental treatment which, in the
absence of consent, could constitute a trespass to the person, is effective
as if the minor were of full age. It should be noted that subsection 3 of
the 1969 Act confuses the issue, using wording designed to sustain the
common law rights of legal minors. It states: "Nothing in this Section
should be construed as making ineffective any consent which would
have been effective if the Section had not been enacted." Thus, when
patients are over 16 years of age, parents cannot override their
consent to treatment, although of course, when they are unable to
give consent, for example when in need of life-saving procedures,
it will be good practice for doctors to obtain agreement, wherever
possible, from the legal guardians. It will also be appropriate in
general for parents and guardians to be involved, with the young
person's consent, in treatment plans made on his or her behalf.

The legislation gives no guidance on informal treatment of young
people under 16 years of age. The common law and the judgement, on
appeal to the House of Lords, in *Gillick* v. *West Norfolk* and *Wisbech
Health Authority* and the *DHSS* [1985] AC 112 are relevant.

The Gillick judgement made three points.

(a) Parental powers are for the protection of the child.
(b) Parental powers dwindle as the child matures (Lord Scarman
    said, "Parental rights yield to the child's right to make his
    own decisions when he reaches sufficient understanding and
    intelligence to be capable of making up his own mind on the
    matter requiring decision.").
(c) Parental powers depend on the understanding of the individual
    child, not on any fixed age.

Lord Scarman said:

> The common law has never treated rights as sovereign or beyond
> review and control. Nor has our law ever treated the child as other
> than a person with capacities and rights recognised by law. Parental
> rights are derived from parental duty and exist only so long as they
> are needed for the protection of the child. The law relating to
> parent and child is concerned with the problems of the growth
> and maturity of human personality. If the law should impose upon
> the process of 'growing up' the fixed limits where nature knows

only a continuous process, the price would be artificiality and a lack of realism in an area where the law must be sensitive to human development and social change.

Thus young people under 16 years of age may be able to consent to psychiatric treatment or to refuse it and the doctor treating them has a responsibility to form a judgement upon their capacity to do this.

Detained patients

The mental health legislation gives no guidance to the detention of minor patients, being enacted without lower age limits save in respect of guardianship (discussed below). Young people under 18 years of age therefore may be detained under the relevant section of the Mental Health Act 1983. This happens infrequently in practice but psychiatrists concerned with these decisions must be familiar with the legislation and the memorandum on Parts I–VI, VIII and X of the Act (see Department of Health and Social Security, 1983*b*), and its updates as these occur.

In a second specific reference to age limits, sections 7–11 of the Act describe guardianship, which allows a patient who has attained the age of 16 years to be placed under the supervision of a guardian approved by a department of social services. The application is made to the social services authority and must be based on medical recommendations from two doctors (one approved), each of whom has examined the patient with no more than five days having elapsed between these examinations. The powers of the guardian are:

(a) to require the patient to reside at a specified place
(b) to require the patient to attend at specific places and times for medical treatment, occupation, education or training
(c) to require access to a patient to be given at the patient's residence to any doctor, approved social worker or other specified person.

The guardian has no power to make the patient accept the treatment and guardianship does not allow detention under secure conditions.

Mentally abnormal offenders

There is no reference to age limits in the mental health legislation but where legal minors are involved in criminal offences, and psychiatric opinions or reports are sought concerning them, it is important to cross-check with relevant legislation concerning criminal justice.

Section 35: Remand to hospital for report: empowers either a magistrates' court or a crown court to remand an accused person, awaiting trial, and accused of an imprisonable offence or awaiting sentence, to a specified hospital for a report.

Section 36: Remand for treatment: empowers a crown court to remand an accused person to a specified hospital for treatment.

Section 37: Hospital and guardianship orders: applies only to individuals found guilty of an imprisonable offence except murder.

These sections may apply to children and young people as defined in child care legislation. The term 'sentenced to prison' applies to young people subject to youth custody or detention orders. The above sections therefore may apply to young people under 17 years of age or to young people under 14 tried and sentenced with an adult.

Discussion

Hoggett (1990) has pointed out that mental health legislation has rarely been used for young people under 16 years of age. It has been supposed that the power to admit a child to hospital is within the right of the parent, the child being subject to parental control. Hoggett comments, with reference to the rights of parents to volunteer their children for psychiatric treatment, "These principles leave a great deal of discretion in the hands of parents and doctors. There is every reason to believe that parents of handicapped or mentally disturbed children find it hard to put their children's interests first all the time." The Children Act 1989, with its emphasis on the obligation to ascertain the views of the child, and recent work on the competence of children as witnesses (Spencer & Flin, 1993) emphasise the need, not just for the child's informed consent to health procedures, but for the physician, and perhaps in particular the child and adolescent psychiatrist, to make a sensitive and informed assessment of the child's comprehension of the issues involved. Richard White discusses child assessment orders on page 112.

Ethically and legally considerable discretion remains in the hands of physicians. Where they are managing scarce NHS resources, they are bound by an ethical code and by the common law; this may be less inadequate than where, as has been described in the USA (Krisberg & Schwartz, 1983; Schwartz *et al*, 1984), the availability of private psychiatric facilities and insurance paid for by parents may enable the admission, on parental authority, of young people, without explicit assessment and discussion of their legal rights, to psychiatric institutions. In England, however, the Gillick judgement may go some way towards counterbalancing this situation. Guidance, regulations and codes of practice may be broken in public or private practice and they require monitoring across jurisdictions and in differing systems of service provision.

In summary, young people over 16 years have the right to consent to or to refuse treatment, but they may be overruled by a person exercising parental responsibility or by the court. Those under 16 may have such rights according to their age and understanding (to be judged by the physician consulted), but they may also be overruled by a person exercising parental responsibility or by the court. It will normally be good practice for the psychiatrist to consult parents and guardians and to obtain their consent to, and involvement in, the treatment of young people. However, where the latter do not agree with advice given, it may be appropriate to consider child protection issues or the applicability of mental health legislation. If the latter legislation is used, parents and guardians will take on the role of nearest relative, with regard, where relevant, to court decisions concerning wardship, care proceedings or custody decisions (see Richardson & Harris-Hendriks, 1996).

Check-list

(a) (i) What is the age of the child concerned?
     (ii) Is the child of an age and understanding to consent to examination or treatment and if so, does he or she give such consent?
(b) (i) Who is the legal guardian(s)?
     (ii) Do the guardians agree to the provision of psychiatric services to the child?
(c) (i) Is the child subject to judicial proceedings?
     (ii) Does a court, its representative, or the child's solicitor, agree to or request psychiatric assessment?
(d) If the answer to any of the secondary questions is in the negative, consider further consultation (including obtaining, if possible, legal advice) and the implications and possible use of the mental health legislation.

Secure accommodation

The body of law in the Children and Young Persons Act (England and Wales) 1969 was modified by the Criminal Justice Act 1982. The 1969 Act seemed to shift the emphasis in dealing with juvenile offenders from the magistrates' courts, which until then had power to determine the disposal of a child. Instead, those children found guilty by a court could, among the options available, be committed to the care of a local authority and specific decisions about the child's placement and treatment would be made by professional social workers. This choice of disposal included the use of 'secure accommodation'.

During the 1970s, along with an increasing use of secure accommodation within the prison system (detention centre and youth custody, formerly known as borstal training) came the development of 'secure units', monitored and managed by the local authority departments of social services. These are now subject to inspection by Social Services Inspectorates of the Department of Health and the Welsh Office.

The Criminal Justice Act 1982 took account of the European Court of Human Rights, in recognising that it was not appropriate or proper that any person should be placed in secure accommodation by administrative process and in the absence of a judicial hearing. The Criminal Justice and Public Order Act 1994 has increased the maximum sentence for an offender via a Secure Training Order as described in the previous chapter.

The Children Act 1989 sets out in detail the conditions under which children may be detained.

In summary, children must be brought before a magistrates' court within three days of being placed by a local authority in secure accommodation. The court decides:

(a) (i) whether they have a history of absconding and are likely to abscond from any other description of accommodation; and

   (ii) if they abscond, whether they are likely to suffer significant harm; or

(b) if they are kept in any other description of accommodation, whether they are likely to injure themselves or other persons.

The court should make a Secure Accommodation Order (for up to three months at a time) if the criteria apply. It is unlawful for the liberty of a child in care to be restricted unless one of these criteria is met.

It should be noted however that these regulations may enable the locking up of young people under 18 years of age who have not committed any crime for which they might have received a custodial sentence, had they reached the age of full majority. This encapsulates yet again a concern by society on behalf of children who are seen as in need of receiving care and protection and who, paradoxically, may be seen as requiring to be locked up in order that they may be protected. In contrast to mental health legislation, there is no requirement to make the case for the 'treatability' of the young person. The regulations recently have been amended to allow secure accommodation to be provided by private organisations.

These regulations tend to lead towards the provision of secure accommodation for a distinct group of young people: absconders (who may well be reflecting the institution from which they abscond rather than any internal pathology), children at risk of self-damage, and children in 'moral danger'. This is a different, although overlapping, group from those young people who end up in custodial institutions because they are on remand or have been convicted of offences to which a custodial response is seen as appropriate. They also overlap with the group of young people referred for special education and admitted to psychiatric hospitals (Stewart & Tutt, 1988).

Child and adolescent psychiatrists may be drawn into this debate both in respect of individual children, when asked to provide expert evidence to magistrates' courts, and when asked to provide consultation to institutions where young people are contained. It is essential that they become aware of the complex legal and ethical dilemmas relevant to work in this field.

Section II Richard White
Child welfare law

The Children Act 1989, implemented on 14 October 1991, introduced comprehensive changes to legislation in England and Wales affecting the welfare of children. It extends to the private law, that is law affecting arrangements within the family, and to the public law, that is involving the family and the state, primarily through local authorities (White *et al*, 1995).

Central themes of the legislation are the autonomy of the family through the exercise of parental responsibility, the provision of services by the local authority, in particular to support families whose children are in need, and protection of children who may be suffering or likely to suffer significant harm. An innovation of the Act is the way in which these different strands are intertwined, so that private law orders can be made in public law proceedings and public law applications can be made in private law proceedings.

The Act contains specific provisions (sections 2–5) concerning parental responsibility. This is something which parents have and, short of adoption (or freeing for adoption), do not lose. The father of a non-marital child can acquire parental responsibility by court order or by agreement with the mother; a testamentary guardian appointed by a parent may act from the death of that person or the surviving spouse.

As a child gets older, the power to exercise parental responsibility dwindles. Thus a child who is of sufficient understanding to make an informed decision may be capable of giving consent to examination or treatment, although the parent or other person having parental responsibility can still give consent on behalf of the child. (See Re *R (A Minor) (Wardship: Medical Treatment)* [1992] Fam 11, Court of Appeal.)

Welfare of the child

When a court determines a question with respect to the upbringing of a child, his or her welfare shall be the court's paramount consideration. Four additional points concerning the welfare of the child need to be considered.

(a) The court is required in public and private law proceedings to establish a timetable and give directions for the expeditious handling of the case, because the court must have regard to the general principle that any delay is likely to prejudice the welfare of the child. This will have implications on attendance at court and the speed with which reports for court will have to be prepared.

(b) There is a check-list to be applied in some opposed private law applications and in care proceedings. The court will be well briefed on this list and so any person giving evidence to the court would be well advised to ensure that their evidence takes account of the check-list. By section 1(3), the court must have regard to:

(i) the ascertainable wishes and feelings of the child (considered in the light of his or her age and understanding)
(ii) the child's physical, emotional and educational needs
(iii) the likely effect on the child of any change in circumstances
(iv) the child's age, gender, background and any characteristics which the court considers relevant
(v) any harm which the child has suffered or is at risk of suffering
(vi) how capable each of the parents is, and any other person in relation to whom the court considers the question to be relevant, of meeting the child's needs
(vii) the range of powers available to the court in the proceedings in question.

(c) One of the most fundamental principles in the new legislation comes under section 1(5), which states that "where a court is considering whether or not to make one or more orders under this Act with respect to a child, it shall not make the order unless it considers that doing so would be better for the child than making no order at all". In other words, contrary to pre-Children Act practice, the court will not be disposed to make any order unless a specific reason is established.

(d) In care proceedings the local authority, in addition to the check-list, must bear in mind that, if it is seeking a care order, it is dealing with a case where it is proposing to look after the child. This applies under section 22(4) and (5), by which the local authority is required, as far as reasonably practicable, to ascertain and give due consideration to the wishes and feelings of the child (having regard to age and understanding), the parents or any other person who has parental responsibility, and any other person the authority considers relevant. It must also give due consideration to the child's religious persuasion, racial origin, and cultural and linguistic background.

Section 8 orders

The most important of the private law orders are known as section 8 orders. These are (see Glossary (pp. 203–208) for definitions):

residence order (note that by section 12 if the order is made in favour of any person who is not a parent or guardian, that person shall have parental responsibility for the duration of the order)
contact order
prohibited steps order
specific issue order

By section 11(7) of the Act a section 8 order may:

(a) contain directions about how it is to be carried into effect
(b) impose directions which must be complied with by any person
  (i) in whose favour the order is made
  (ii) who is a parent of the child concerned
  (iii) who is not a parent but who has parental responsibility or
  (iv) with whom the child is living and to whom the conditions are expressed to apply
(c) be made to have effect for a specified period or contain provisions which are to have effect for a specified period
(d) make such incidental, supplemental or consequential provision as the court thinks fit.

Because by section 1(3) the court must consider the range of orders available under the Act, section 8 orders can be made in care proceedings, whether or not the threshold criteria (described below) are satisfied. It is possible that the courts will seek to exercise control through the use of these orders applying the principles in section 1 of the Act. They may prefer not to make a care order by which the local authority acquires parental responsibility, even though the threshold criteria are satisfied. Judicious use of section 8 orders and section 11(7) directions and/or conditions may provide a suitable alternative. Courts may not make a care order and a section 8 order at the same time.

Child protection

In relation to child protection, doctors may be involved in care proceedings under section 31, or applications for a child assessment order under section 43, or emergency protection under section 44. The local authority has duties to investigate suspicion of significant harm. It is entitled to expect the cooperation of other agencies with responsibilities for children. If it cannot get parental cooperation, it may wish to seek court assistance. This may involve seeking a child assessment order with the child remaining at home, but emergency removal may sometimes be necessary.

Care proceedings

Application to the court for a care or supervision order may be made only by a local authority or an authorised person, which is defined by section 31(9) as the National Society for the Prevention of Cruelty to Children (NSPCC) and any of its officers or any other person authorised by the Secretary of State, of which there are none as yet. Thus applications may no longer be made by the police, and an education authority is limited to making an application for an education supervision order under section 36.

Criteria for the court

The court may make a care order or a supervision order, in respect of a child under 17 (or 16 if married), only if it is satisfied that:

  (a) the child concerned is suffering significant harm, or is likely to suffer significant harm; and
  (b) the harm or likelihood of harm is attributable to:
      (i)   the care given to the child, or likely to be given to him or her if the order were not made, not being what it would be reasonable to expect a parent to give to the child; or
      (ii) the child's being beyond parental control (section 31(2)).

The court has to consider the question of whether a child is suffering significant harm at the time when the local authority acts to protect the child: Re *M. (A Minor) (Care Order: Significant Harm)* [1994] 2 AC 424. Whether harm is likely is a matter for the court. If the application is based on the likelihood that the child will suffer significant harm on the grounds that a previous child has been harmed, the authority must satisfy the court of those facts on the balance of probabilities, and not solely that there is a reasonable prospect overall that the child will suffer harm. The court must be satisfied that the evidence is cogent and commensurate with the seriousness of the allegations. (See Re *H (Threshold Criteria) (Standard of Proof)* [1996] 1 FLR 80.)

The court must also

(a) apply the principles contained in section 1
(b) have regard to the check-list in section 1(3), and
(c) not make an order unless it considers that doing so would be better for the child than making no order at all.

Thus the threshold criteria are not in themselves grounds or reasons for making a care or supervision order. The court will want to know what plans the authority has if the child is committed to care, whether these could be carried out if the child was accommodated without a care order, and why services to the family provided under Part III of the Act would not sufficiently protect the child.

Effect of a care order

Making a care order discharges any section 8 order and brings wardship to an end (section 91). The child must be received and kept in care while the order is in force. The authority has parental responsibility, but the parent does not cease to have parental responsibility solely because some other person acquires it. The local authority has the power to determine the extent to which a parent or guardian may meet his or her parental responsibility insofar as it is necessary to do so to safeguard or promote the child's welfare.

The implication of the continuation of the responsibility of the parent is that the authority must continue to work with the parent. This has created a new emphasis which has required local authorities to seek to work in partnership with parents before and after a care order is made.

Supervision

Under a supervision order the court may by Schedule 3 require the supervised child to comply with any directions given from time to time by the supervisor which require the child to:

(a) live at a place or places specified in the directions for a specified period or periods
(b) present himself or herself to a specified person at a place and on a day specified
(c) participate in specified activities.

The supervisor shall decide whether and to what extent and in what form he or she shall exercise this power. This does not confer on the supervisor power to direct medical or psychiatric examination or treatment. The court may include a requirement in a supervision order, with the consent of and in relation to a 'responsible person' (that is a person with parental responsibility or with whom the child is living), that the responsible person takes all reasonable steps to ensure that the child complies with any direction given by the supervisor, that he or she takes all reasonable steps to ensure that the child complies with any requirement in relation to psychiatric and medical examination or treatment, and that he or she complies with the supervisor's directions on attending at a specified place.

A supervision order (but not an interim supervision order) may require the supervised child to:

(a) submit to a medical or psychiatric examination
(b) submit to such an examination from time to time as directed by the supervisor
(c) submit to specified treatment in relation to a mental or physical condition.

Schedule 3 paragraphs 4 and 5 contain detailed provisions which have to be satisfied before a requirement can be imposed. Both these provisions are made subject to the proviso that a child of sufficient understanding to make an informed decision must consent to the inclusion of the requirement. Thus, child and adolescent psychiatrists, if asked to provide diagnosis or treatment within the framework of a supervision order, must still consider the child's capacity to give or withhold consent to treatment and also the need for the informed involvement of parents, guardians and other key family workers and professionals. It will be appropriate for the psychiatrist to advise the court on the feasibility of making an order that 'requires' psychiatric assessment.

Interim measures

If the court is satisfied that there are reasonable grounds for believing that the threshold criteria are satisfied, it may make an interim care order or an interim supervision order. They may be made initially for up to eight weeks and thereafter for four weeks.

If an interim residence order under section 8 is made in care proceedings, there is a presumption that an interim supervision order should also be made. The court must also apply the overriding principles in section 1 that the welfare of the child is paramount and that an order should only be made if it is better for the child than making no order.

Directions on interim applications

Where the court makes an interim care or supervision order, it may give such directions as it considers appropriate with regard to medical or psychiatric examination or other assessment of the child and may direct that no examination or assessment is to take place at all or unless the court directs. If the child is of sufficient understanding to make an informed decision he or she may refuse to submit to an examination or assessment.

Discharge of a care order

Discharge of a care order may be achieved by an application under section 39, but if a person wishes to acquire parental responsibility he or she should seek a residence order under section 8, the making of which would end the care order.

Appeal

All parties to proceedings may appeal against the making of an order. Pending an appeal the court may make interim orders subject to such directions as it sees fit.

Contact with children in care

Section 34(1) requires the local authority to allow a child who is subject to a care order (including an interim care order) reasonable contact with:

(a) the parents or guardian
(b) a person in whose favour there was a residence order immediately before the making of the care order
(c) a person who had the care of the child by virtue of an order under the inherent jurisdiction of the High Court.

Although there is no specific provision, all parties should expect to reach a written agreement on the terms for contact and other arrangements while the child is in care.

Persons designated in section 34(1) may apply to the court as of right for an order under section 34 with regard to the contact they are to be allowed with the child. Applications may also be made by any person who has obtained the leave of the court. This will enable relatives to seek contact and in most cases they are likely to be granted leave to apply. In some circumstances former foster parents may wish to seek contact. Applications may be made by the local authority or the child for defined contact.

On making a care order, or later, the court may make such order as it considers appropriate as to the contact to be allowed (section 34(1) and (2)). The welfare of the child is the paramount consideration and the other principles in section 1 apply (see above). Such conditions as the court considers appropriate may be attached. This may include restriction of contact to specific periods or places.

Refusal of contact

The local authority or the child may apply for an order authorising the authority to refuse to allow contact between the child and any named person. The child's welfare is the paramount consideration. Although the plans of a local authority, for example, to place a child for adoption, will be taken into account, ultimately the decision as to contact is the responsibility of the court. As a matter of urgency an authority may refuse to allow contact for up to seven days, if it is satisfied that it is necessary to do so in order to safeguard or promote the child's welfare.

Where an applicant has been refused any order under section 34, he or she may not make another such application within six months without the leave of the court. The court may order that no application for any order under the Act may be made by a named person without the leave of the court.

Child assessment orders

The court may make a child assessment order under section 43 on the application of a local authority or authorised person, if it is satisfied that:

(a) the applicant has reasonable cause to suspect that a child is suffering, or is likely to suffer significant harm

(b) an assessment of the state of the child's health or development, or of the way in which the child has been treated, is required to enable the applicant to determine whether or not the child is suffering, or is likely to suffer, significant harm; and

(c) it is unlikely that such an assessment will be made, or be satisfactory, in the absence of a child assessment order.

It is an application made on notice to the parties; it is not intended to be used in an emergency nor as a substitute for an emergency protection order. The child assessment order is appropriate where attempts to achieve an assessment have been frustrated, whereas the emergency protection order suggests a more immediate risk to the child.

The court may make directions relating to the assessment, including directions as to the kind of assessment which is to take place and with what aim, by whom and where it will be carried out, and whether it will be subject to conditions. The child may only be kept away from home in accordance with directions specified in the order, if it is necessary for the purposes of the assessment and for such period or periods as specified in the order.

Any person who is in a position to produce the child is under a duty to produce him or her to the person named in the order and to comply with such directions relating to the assessment of the child as may be specified in the order. The order authorises any person carrying out the assessment, or any part of it, to do so in accordance with the order.

If the child is of sufficient understanding to make an informed decision, he or she may refuse to submit to a medical or psychiatric examination or other assessment, even though the court has made an order.

Emergency protection order

The court may make an emergency protection order under section 44(1)(a) on the application of any person if it is satisfied that there is reasonable cause to believe that the child is likely to suffer significant harm if the child:

    (a) is not removed to accommodation provided by or on behalf of the applicant, or

    (b) does not remain in the place where he or she is being accommodated.

Section 1 applies. Alternatives must be considered, such as accommodation of the child, departure of the person causing the danger to the child, or placement with friends or relatives.

Significant harm must be likely. Evidence of harm which was occurring at the time of the application or has occurred in the past is not sufficient unless it indicates that harm is likely to occur.

A local authority may also apply for an order under section 44(1)(b) where it is making inquiries because it has reasonable cause to suspect that a child is suffering, or is likely to suffer, significant harm, and those inquiries are being frustrated by access to the child being unreasonably refused to a person authorised to seek access and it has reasonable cause to believe that access to the child is required as a matter of urgency. An important part of the test will obviously be whether the refusal to allow the child to be seen is unreasonable. The court will need to know what efforts have been made to see the child and what responses have been made by the child's caretakers.

The court may take account of any statement contained in any report made to the court in the course of, or in connection with, the hearing or any evidence given during the hearing, which is in the opinion of the court relevant to the application. This enables the court to give proper weight to hearsay, opinions, health visiting or social work records and medical reports, and will avoid the need for attendance at court by a doctor at this stage. The provision of advice and reports, in particular concerning contact and the need for a medical or psychiatric examination or assessment and related directions likely to be made by the court, will be important.

Effect

An emergency protection order operates as a direction to any person who is in a position to do so to comply with any request to produce the child to the applicant and authorises removal to or prevention of removal from accommodation provided by or on behalf of the applicant. If the applicant is refused entry, the court may issue a warrant authorising a constable to assist in the execution of the order using reasonable force if necessary.

The court may include a requirement under section 44(a) providing for a person to be excluded from a home in which he is living with a child. The grounds for an emergency protection order must be satisfied and the court must be satisfied that if the requirement is imposed the child will not be likely to suffer significant harm.

An emergency protection order gives the applicant parental responsibility for the child, but this is limited insofar as the applicant shall only exercise the power to remove or prevent removal in order to safeguard and promote the welfare of the child. If an applicant gains access and finds that the child is not harmed or likely to be harmed, the child may not be removed. If during the order a return home to a parent or other connected person appears to be safe, then the applicant is required to carry that out, although the child may be removed again if a change in circumstances makes it necessary.

Duration of emergency protection order

The order may be granted for up to eight days, although the court may order one extension for up to seven days if it has reasonable cause to believe that the child is likely to suffer significant harm if the order is not extended (section 45).

There is no appeal against matters connected with an emergency protection order, but an application to discharge the order may be heard between three and eight days after it was made, by the child, a parent, any other person with parental responsibility or any person with whom the child was living immediately before the making of the order, except where that person was present at or given notice of the hearing. Any directions (see below) the court gives may also be the subject of an application to vary.

Contact during emergency protection order

The applicant must allow the child reasonable contact, during the period of an order, subject to the directions of the court, with parents, any other person with parental responsibility, any person with whom the child was living immediately before the order, any person in whose favour there is a contact order in relation to the child and any person acting on behalf of those persons.

The court may (not must), on making the order, and at any time while it is in force, give such directions as it considers appropriate in relation to contact between the child and any named person. The court may give directions as to contact that is or is not to be allowed between the child and any named person, and may impose conditions.

Medical or psychiatric examination or assessment

The court may give directions as to a medical or psychiatric examination or other assessment of the child, and it is specifically provided that the court may direct that there is to be no examination or no examination unless the court directs otherwise. The child may refuse to submit to an examination or other assessment if he or she is of sufficient understanding to make an informed decision, even though the court has ordered it. It will be an important decision for the doctor as to the understanding of the child.

Police protection

The police also have powers under section 46 to take a child into police protection for up to 72 hours. They do not acquire parental responsibility but do have a duty to do what is reasonable in all the circumstances of the case for the purpose of safeguarding or promoting the child's welfare. Whether this is sufficient to authorise a medical examination remains unclear and may require further clarification.

Local authority services

Part III of the 1989 Act places a general duty on local authorities to safeguard and promote the welfare of children in their area who are in need and, so far as is consistent with that duty, to promote the upbringing of such children by their families by providing a range and level of services appropriate to those children's needs (section 17(1)).

Children, that is persons under 18 years, are in need if they are unlikely to achieve or maintain, or to have the opportunity of achieving or maintaining, a reasonable standard of health or development without the provision for them of services by a local authority under Part III, or if their health or development is likely to be significantly impaired or further impaired, without the provision for them of such services, or if they are disabled (section 17(10)).

A child is disabled if blind, deaf or dumb or suffering from mental disorder of any kind or if substantially and permanently disabled by illness, injury or congenital deformity or such other disability as may be prescribed (section 17(11)). By this provision disabled children are brought into the mainstream of legislation and entitled to the same services as other children.

Local authorities are given a number of duties in relation to what might broadly be described as family support mechanisms. They should make provision for advice, guidance, counselling and home help. They also have duties to provide such day care as is appropriate and to provide accommodation for children in certain circumstances.

The provision of accommodation as a service to the family replaces the old-style 'voluntary care'. The local authority has no parental responsibility for the child but does have certain duties, as it is looking after the child. The parent can remove the child from accommodation at will. Parents should, however, work in partnership with the local authority in accordance with agreed arrangements to ensure that accommodation, as with other services, benefits the child.

Long-term substitute care

A local authority has a duty under section 23 of the Children Act 1989 to provide accommodation and maintenance for children it is looking after. It may do this by placing children with the parents, although it is an unlikely first step. If a care order is in force, the authority must act in accordance with the Accommodation of Children with Parents etc. Regulations 1991, which require inquiries to be made about the parents.

The authority may also place the child with foster parents, or in a children's home or by making such other arrangements as seem appropriate. Residential provision is less likely for a younger child.

Where people other than the birth parents have the long-term care of a child, they will probably wish to have some kind of security to reflect their responsibility as substitute parents. If they are fostering the child for a local authority this may be sufficient on a short-term basis, or even a longer-term basis for an older child. If the foster parents want parental responsibility themselves, they will have to consider seeking a residence order under section 8 (see above) or an adoption order.

If foster parents seek a residence order, they will have to bear in mind that the parent continues to have parental responsibility, so that while the substitute carers acquire parental responsibility, they will effectively have to share it with the parents.

Adoption

An adoption bill was published in 1996 which would introduce numerous changes to adoption legislation but it is unlikely to be implemented at an early date. Until then, most adoption provisions are contained in the Adoption Act 1976, a statute which consolidates previous enactments. (All statutory references are to the 1976 Act unless otherwise stated.) These regulate the activities of adoption agencies, that is local authorities or approved adoption societies, when a child is placed with them for adoption or when they decide that a child in their care should be considered for adoption.

The statutory duty set out in section 6 is of first importance:

> In reaching any decision relating to the adoption of a child, a court or adoption agency shall have regard to all the circumstances, first consideration being given to the need to safeguard and promote the welfare of the child throughout his childhood; and shall so far as practicable ascertain the wishes and feelings of the child regarding the decision and give due consideration to them, having regard to his age and understanding.

Agency placements

Under the Act a local authority has a duty to provide a com-prehensive adoption service and the Adoption Agencies Regulations

1983 set out how this should be carried out in any particular case. This includes duties to children and their parents, duties to prospective adopters and duties in respect of a proposed placement. An agency is required to set up a panel to carry out certain of its functions.

An agency may pay an adoption allowance in accordance with regulations made under section 57A of the Adoption Act 1976. This is likely to be limited to children with special needs, where there is disability or where a sibling group is to be adopted.

An adoption order vests parental responsibility relating to a child in the adopters and from the making of the order extinguishes the parental responsibility of any person who had such responsibility immediately before the making of the order. The order can be made only by an authorised court and application may be made to the magistrates' court, county court or High Court, but contested cases should not be heard in the magistrates' court.

The court cannot make the order unless the child is free for adoption (see below) or the parents agree or there are grounds for dispensing with the agreement of the parents.

Qualified individuals (a married couple or a single person) may apply in respect of a child living with them. In the case of a placement by an adoption agency or in pursuance of a High Court order or where one of the applicants is a relative, an order cannot be made until the child is at least 19 weeks old and has lived with the applicants for at least 13 weeks. In other cases (i.e. private placements) an order cannot be made until the child is at least 12 months old and has lived with the applicants (or one of them) for 12 months.

Freeing order

An adoption agency may apply to the court for an order freeing the child for adoption. Such an order will vest the parental responsibility in the agency, in the expectation that an adoption order will be made later. A freeing order cannot be made unless the court is satisfied that the parents agree to the making of the order or that there are grounds for dispensing with their agreement.

This order has advantages: for the parents – they can, if they wish, be relieved of their responsibilities at an early stage; for the adopters – they can take the child secure in the knowledge that the question of parental agreement has already been dealt with.

There are disadvantages, because there may still be delay in court proceedings during which the parent may withdraw agreement, and if a parent does not agree the outcome is uncertain. The adoption agency has to take a difficult decision as to whether the welfare of the child requires the child to be placed with prospective adopters before the freeing order is made, even though the outcome of the application is uncertain.

In practice most adoption agencies seem to be using the freeing provisions only in limited circumstances, examples of which are:

(a) where the parent will have nothing further to do with the child, but it is unlikely that the child will be placed quickly (even then, because of resources, many agencies will feel that the separate court application is not worthwhile)
(b) where the question of placement for adoption is very contentious, and the child cannot be placed until it is resolved
(c) where there is a desire not to involve the prospective adopters with a contested application.

Agreement

The agreement of each parent or guardian must be given freely and unconditionally and with full understanding of what is involved, either to the adoption order itself or to the freeing order. ('Parent or guardian' does not include an unmarried father unless he has parental responsibility under section 4 of the Children Act 1989.) Without agreement an order may be made only if there are grounds for dispensing with agreement.

Dispensation with parental agreement

If a person whose agreement is required refuses to give it, the court may dispense with the agreement where the person:

(a) cannot be found or is incapable of giving agreement
(b) withholds agreement unreasonably
(c) fails to discharge parental obligations or ill-treats the child in various specified ways.

Whether agreement is withheld reasonably is a vital question in contested adoptions and has been considered in numerous legal decisions since the leading case of Re *W (An Infant)* [1971] AC 682. The court has to consider the position at the time of the hearing. The court must apply an objective test and consider what a reasonable parent in the position of the actual parent would do in the circumstances. The court cannot simply substitute its own view for that of the parent. It must consider whether a parental veto comes within the band of possible reasonable decisions and not whether it is right or mistaken. The welfare of the child must be taken into account, since the reasonable parent gives great weight to it. The claims of the natural parents and the adopting family must also be taken into account.

There are other specific issues which the courts have had to take into account in recent cases:

(a) how the long-term security of the child will best be promoted;
(b) whether contact with the parent is important for the child and if so to what extent (the more intense the contact, the less likely and perhaps less appropriate is adoption, and the less likely it is that the court can find that a parent is withholding agreement unreasonably);
(c) whether there are ethnic or religious factors, which may enable a parent to withhold agreement reasonably.

In family placements

Step-parents or relatives may apply to adopt a child. If there have been divorce proceedings, step-parents may have to return to the divorce court for variation of the custody or residence order. Relatives should also consider whether adoption or a residence order is the better alternative.

Adoption contact register

Section 51A of the Adoption Act 1976 requires the Registrar-General to register the name and address of any adopted person over 18, and whose birth record is kept by the Registrar-General, who gives notice that he or she wishes to contact a relative. The Registrar-General is also required to register the name and address of a relative (defined as a person who is related to the adopted person by blood, including half-blood, or marriage) of an adopted person who is over 18 and has such information as is necessary to enable a record of the adopted person's birth to be obtained.

The Registrar-General then has to transmit to the registered adopted person the name and address of any registered relative. The address given can be an address at or through which the person concerned may be contacted. The legislation contains no provision for counselling.

Alternatives to adoption

In all adoption applications the alternatives to adoption should be carefully considered in any report. The court has power to make section 8 orders (see above) instead of, and in some circumstances in addition to, an adoption order.

Adoption Bill 1996

If current proposals are enacted local authorities will have to obtain a placement order from a court before a child may be placed for adoption: unless the child is not subject to a care order and the parents, or those with parental authority, give consent. As ever, practitioners need to remain abreast of legislative change.

The courts

There are a number of courts which deal with matters relating to children, and in which a child and adolescent psychiatrist may have to appear to give evidence or present a report.

Youth court

This court now deals solely with juvenile offenders.

Magistrates' court

With the advent of the Children Act 1989 a 'family panel' of magistrates will have powers to deal with 'family proceedings' in the 'family proceedings court'. Care proceedings must be started in that court, although they may be allocated to a higher court. Magistrates do not have jurisdiction in relation to divorce, wardship and the inherent jurisdiction of the High Court, child abduction, and some cases of domestic violence. They do have jurisdiction to make orders in respect of children, including orders under section 8 of the 1989 Act (see above), maintenance, adoption and domestic violence between spouses.

The family proceedings court will have a lay bench of two or three magistrates, sitting with a justices' clerk. A stipendiary magistrate may sometimes sit. Magistrates are referred to as 'Sir' or 'Madam' or 'Your Worships'.

County court

In this court a judge, who is a barrister or solicitor of at least 10 years' standing, sits alone and is referred to as 'Your Honour'. He or she may deal with a wide range of civil matters. Following implementation of the Children Act, family cases are dealt with at a family hearing centre or a care centre, depending on the nature of the case. Care proceedings allocated from the magistrates' court because of their complexity will be heard at a limited number of nation-wide care centres by judges who have had special training for the purpose. The wider range of orders available under the Act and other matters such as divorce and nullity, domestic violence and adoption are heard at a family hearing centre.

As to the District Judges, depending on the area, they sit in the county court and may additionally sit in the High Court. In the provinces they have limited jurisdiction to hear some substantive matters in private law and give directions in public law cases. At the Principal Registry of the Family Division there are a number of District Judges who give directions, make interim orders but are also authorised to hear care proceedings. They are addressed as 'Sir' or 'Madam'.

Authorised clerks in family proceedings courts have power to give directions in care proceedings on unopposed matters.

High Court

This court has a number of divisions. Family matters are dealt with in the Family Division either at the Royal Courts of Justice in the Strand in London or at a district registry. There are 17 Family Division judges, but the Lord Chancellor also appoints deputy judges to sit from time to time. A local county court judge may be appointed to act as a deputy High Court judge. High Court judges sit alone to hear complex cases under the Children Act and in adoption, wardship, and the inherent jurisdiction and appeals from the magistrates' court. Certain appeals are to the Divisional Court when two judges will sit together. High Court judges are called 'My Lord' or 'My Lady' (see also Chapter 4).

Court of Appeal

Appeals from the High Court and county court go to the Court of Appeal and are heard by two or three Lords Justices of Appeal. There is not always an automatic right of appeal and the leave of the judge may be necessary. Even where there is an automatic right, legal practitioners are warned not to pursue appeals without clear grounds for doing so. Witnesses do not usually give evidence.

House of Lords

This is the final court of appeal in the United Kingdom and will only hear cases where there is an issue of public importance. Cases are heard before five Law Lords. Witnesses do not give evidence.

The High Court, Court of Appeal and the House of Lords are Courts of Record. Each can establish legal precedent which is binding on courts lower than itself. The European Court of Human Rights in Strasbourg is a final court of appeal.

Wardship

Which children?

Any child under the age of 18 who is in England and Wales may be made a ward of court, although its use is now rare. This is subject only to the restriction that if the child is the subject of proceedings in Scotland or Northern Ireland, the court may only make an order if it considers there is an emergency.

Procedure

There is a very simple procedure for making a child a ward of court. Any person can attend at a registry of the High Court (in London, First Avenue House in Holborn), complete some forms and pay the court fee (currently £100.00). A child becomes a ward as soon as the summons is issued and remains so for 21 days without any further action. An applicant must show an 'interest' in the child and if the court staff are doubtful as to the propriety of the application the matter will be referred to a recorder or deputy judge. Subject to this a summons will be issued together with a notice of wardship. This form states that "without the leave of the Court the Ward may not marry or go outside England and Wales nor should there be any material change in the arrangements for welfare, care and control or education without said leave."

In the event of an emergency, applications for court orders may be made to the registrar of the day (in London) or for more serious matters to the applications judge. A party will be able to make representation at any hearings in relation to the ward. Evidence will usually be filed on affidavit, which may be supplemented or cross-examined orally.

Parties

Anyone may be a party to wardship proceedings with the consent of the court. However, the child will not automatically be made a party, but may be joined if he or she is old enough to express an opinion or if there is a point of law or public importance at issue. If the child is made a party he or she must be represented by a guardian ad litem, and usually this will be the Official Solicitor.

Position following implementation of the Children Act 1989

The 1989 Act makes the use of wardship in the context of private law less necessary because many of the courts' powers become available under the statute. The Act considerably limits the use of wardship by local authorities.

It is necessary to distinguish between wardship and powers that the High Court has under its inherent jurisdiction. Wardship is the vehicle by which historically the courts have exercised their inherent jurisdiction over children, but immediately the child becomes a ward the principles of the jurisdiction apply. The inherent jurisdiction can be used without wardship to obtain specific orders in certain circumstances.

Section 100 of the 1989 Act provides:

(a) no child may be in care and a ward of court;
(b) no order may be made committing a child to care or supervision or requiring him or her to be accommodated under the inherent jurisdiction;
(c) no order may be made to confer on a local authority power to decide an issue of parental responsibility;
(d) the inherent jurisdiction may not be used unless the court has given leave for the application, which can only be given if the result sought could not be achieved by other means (e.g. a section 8 order) and there is reasonable cause to believe the child is likely to suffer significant harm if the inherent jurisdiction is not exercised. There has been very limited use of the provision and so its scope remains uncertain.

Principles of the jurisdiction

The central principle is that the welfare of the child is the paramount consideration, although if the child is subject to immigration procedures, the court will not allow wardship to be used to circumvent the statutory provisions, and will therefore decline to make any orders in respect of the child.

A second important principle is that no important step in the life of a ward may be taken without the leave of the court. This leads to a requirement to obtain the consent of the court before certain steps are taken in respect of the child. Thus if it is necessary for the child to move from a caretaker or if the child is being placed for adoption, the court's consent is required.

Most important to doctors is to be clear as to the circumstances in which they can exercise their discretion in relation to treatment of the child. It is specifically provided by a Practice Direction that a physical examination of a ward does not require the consent of the court. A psychiatric assessment on the other hand does require the consent of the court and it is considered a most serious contempt of court to undertake an assessment without consent. The courts have frequently restated this principle and practitioners should be on their guard in this respect.

The question of medical treatment is more complex, since there is no precise definition as to what medical treatment should be considered an important step in the life of the child. As a guide it may be considered that if the child has to have a general anaesthetic then this should be considered important, but it should not be assumed from this that all treatment that does not require an anaesthetic can be considered unimportant. Practitioners would be well advised to take legal advice if they are in any doubt.

Doctors should also be aware that they are not entitled to look at documents in wardship proceedings (or any other family proceedings) unless the court's consent has been given. It is recommended that the doctor should obtain written confirmation, and in cases of doubt ask to see the court order authorising release of the documents.

Challenge to the local authority

Where a child is in the care of a local authority, the court cannot override any decisions properly taken by that authority, although decisions may be influenced by contact orders under section 34 (see pp. 111–112). Neither wardship nor the inherent jurisdiction may be used for this purpose and it would appear that the only remedy through the courts (as opposed to a complaints procedure, which the authority is required to set up) is judicial review.

This remedy is based on judicial power to control an executive or administrative body where it has acted in breach of statutory duty or taken a decision which no reasonable body could have reached. The remedy is limited in that the court can only require the authority to reconsider its decision.

14 Advice on fees

Whether to charge

National Health Service hospital practitioners are contracted to give a clinical service which includes the examination of and report on a person referred by a medical practitioner, as well as certain other services set out in *Terms and Conditions of Service of Hospital Medical and Dental Staff* (Department of Health, 1994*b*). (Employees of NHS trusts should discuss terms and conditions of service with the relevant managers.) These are called category I services and include "attendance at court hearings as a witness as to fact by a practitioner giving evidence on his own behalf or on behalf of his employing authority in connection with a case with which he is professionally concerned". However, the majority of the work discussed in this book comes into category II (para. 37, *ibid*), for which a fee can be charged. Doctors can charge a fee for providing a medical report on a patient currently under their care if the report would require a special examination or if it would involve an appreciable amount of additional work to prepare it. Attendance at court as a professional or expert witness also comes under category II.

Doctors can also make a charge for work which is not clinical in nature. If a referral is made by a solicitor, or social services department, or a court for an examination of a child in order to help to make a decision about the welfare of the child, a fee can be charged for the examination, the preparation of the report and any subsequent attendance at court as category II work.

It is wise to clarify with the referrer at the beginning whether a referral is being made for NHS diagnosis and treatment or for other purposes. In the latter case it is advisable to ask for a letter of instruction from the referrer in which he or she undertakes to pay the practitioner's reasonable charges.

These considerations do not apply if the provision of reports for the court or a specified social services department forms part of the psychiatrist's contractual duties. The British Medical Association is likely to continue to advise against contracts of this type. Category II work is specifically excluded from the NHS definition of private practice ("Terms and Conditions", para. 40). Fees so obtained *do not* count towards the rule that whole-time practitioners keep their private earnings below 10% of their gross salary. A practitioner is entitled to use NHS time to perform category II work "provided that it would not in the opinion of his employing authority interfere with other hospital activities, or the proper discharge of his contractual duties" (para. 33, *ibid*).

Many NHS practitioners are diffident about making charges. There are several reasons for this:

(a) A conviction that health services should be free at the point of delivery.

(b) Unfamiliarity with charging fees and a reluctance to become involved with 'dirtying one's hands'.

(c) Since these services may be given in time contracted to the NHS, psychiatrists may feel they are being paid twice for the same time.

While respecting these, often deeply held, views the editors consider that proper charges should be made for these non-clinical services for the following reasons:

(a) What is being offered is not a clinical service (although psychiatric advice may benefit the health of the child). If a few practitioners do this work without making a charge, they will become overwhelmed by referrals and this will impair their clinical services. A proper charge should be made which, if desired, can then be donated to their department. The fund should be set up as a charitable trust to avoid income tax. Advice should be sought from the district or trust treasurer.

(b) Doctors are remunerated for their time and expertise (as are all workers). The fact that hospital doctors are paid a salary in the NHS rather than a fee per item of service has removed the direct perception of the value of their individual items of work. If psychiatrists do not value their own work, others will not do so.

(c) Attending court may disrupt the psychiatrist's patient schedules considerably and almost inevitably involves additional out-of-hours work. This out-of-hours NHS work is, of course, not separately remunerated.

Although fees earned are theirs to do with as they wish, some practitioners use fees earned from court work to support research in their departments, to help buy equipment and books, or to allow them and other members of their team to attend conferences, etc. Some consultants choose to make a distinction between work done for their own local authority and for other local authorities and charge only for the latter.

If a psychiatrist is not in full-time NHS practice, and the work is done in non-contracted time, these considerations do not apply and the fees are part of income from private practice. All fees paid directly to the consultant are subject to income tax and it may be helpful to seek advice from an accountant.

Whom to charge

If the request to see a child and prepare a report is made by a solicitor (including the Official Solicitor), social services department or guardian ad litem, the account should go to the referrer. If a judge orders a report, this is usually arranged by the solicitor acting for the local authority, parents or guardian ad litem, and the instructing or lead solicitor should be billed. It is wise to make clear the scale of charges before taking on the case and to deal directly with the legal department of the local authority when the referral comes from social services. Authority for legal aid payments should be obtained, where appropriate, by the instructing solicitor.

How to charge

A separate account should be sent on headed paper, detailing the services given and approximate time spent. The name of the patient should be specified and directions given to whom payment should be made. An example is given below.

What to charge

Fees are a matter for negotiation. In deciding what to charge the following points may be helpful.

(a) Calculate what the time is worth to the NHS, according to salary and the number of hours worked. For example, a consultant psychiatrist on maximum scale earns £x p.a. for a 35-hour week. Annual leave is six weeks, and study leave is two to three weeks, leaving, say, 43 weeks at 35 hours a week. Therefore the hourly rate of pay would be £x/1505 hours.

Royal Sunsetshire Hospital
Department of Child Psychiatry

[Date]
To: Sunsetshire Local Authority Legal Department
or Bloggs & Bloggs, Solicitors
or The Official Solicitor to the Supreme Court

ACCOUNT

To psychiatric examination by Dr Smith of Joe JONES on [date] (2 hours)	£XXX
To perusing the papers.in the case & compiling a psychiatric report (4 hours)	£YYY
To attending court as expert witness on [date] (1 day) including expenses and travelling time	£ZZZ
TOTAL:	£ABC

Please make cheque payable to Dr F. Smith
[or, make cheque payable to Royal Sunsetshire Hospital Research
Fund, and return to Dr F. Smith]

(b) However, for NHS patients, the NHS supplies consulting rooms, secretarial help, stationery, superannuation, insurance, lighting, heating, etc. It pays even when patients cancel. It would be reasonable, therefore, to double the above figure in private cases in order to take into account these overheads, which must be paid for those patients not seen in the NHS.

(c) The Legal Services Division of the Lord Chancellor's Department (Trevelyan House, Great Peter Street, London SW1P 2BY, tel. 0171 210 8772/3) recommends a band of fees that expert witnesses may charge in criminal cases. The figures are available in a regularly updated circular, "Guide to Allowances under Part V of the Costs in Criminal Cases (General) Regulations".

Similar fees to those in criminal cases are also appropriate in civil cases, but if the patient is legally aided then the solicitor must obtain approval in advance for an expert opinion with a maximum fee. A range of fees based on an hourly rate according to seniority, expertise and the type and complexity of the case would seem to be appropriate plus travelling and other expenses. Fees should be revised annually. For court attendance one charges by the half-day rather than the hour. A daily rate would be approximately six times one's hourly rate. Travel expenses and travelling time would be charged additionally, if the court is outside one's catchment area, where relevant.

How to collect

Most solicitors and legal departments of local authorities are prompt in settling accounts. If the patient is legally aided the solicitor can apply to the Law Society Area Legal Aid Office for a payment on account in order to settle professional bills.

If an account has not been paid within two to three months a reminder can be sent; viz:

ACCOUNT

To account rendered on [date]
for professional services to Joe Jones   £ABC etc

Solicitors with large legal aid practices often have to wait a long time for payment and it is sometimes necessary to be patient, but continue to send reminders. Rarely, it will be necessary to apply to the Office for the Supervision of Solicitors (OSS, 8 Dormer Place, Leamington Spa, Warwickshire CV32 5AE; telephone 09126 820082) for help in collecting fees.

Check-list

Do not charge if:

(a) the work is category I
(b) the work is of a clinical nature
(c) the patient is referred by a medical practitioner
(d) the work is part of your contractual duties
(e) you attend court as a witness to fact.

Do charge if:

(a) the work is category II
(b) the patient is referred by solicitor, local authority, court, guardian ad litem, Official Solicitor
(c) preparing a report requires extra consultations or substantial time to peruse papers, etc.
(d) you attend consultations with lawyers, police or guardians
(e) you attend court as an expert or professional witness.

Specimen reports

Introduction

The reports in earlier editions have been replaced by four longer specimen reports. Names and personal details have been changed or omitted to protect confidentiality.

The first, on a private law dispute concerning custody and residence, is set out according to the framework described by Tufnell & Cottrell (1996). (See also, Chapter 3.)

Three additional reports cover, in detail: a child subjected to inter-parental violence, a victim of Munchausen's syndrome by proxy and the child subject of a compensation claim in respect of a head injury. These subsequent reports omit or limit introductory information, the description of documents, copies of letters of instruction and appendices in order to focus on clinical content (sometimes in colloquial detail intended to bring alive the children in the court context), interview techniques or research evidence.

The fourth report is written as recommended in Chapter 10.

Residence and contact

This report, prepared in response to a request, by solicitors representing the parents, for evaluation of written documentation, discusses a dispute between hostile parents whose children, resident with their father, refuse or are reluctant to meet their mother.

Direct evaluation of parents and children is recommended.

Appendices are listed but omitted to save space.

PSYCHIATRIC REPORT

of
Dr [Name] [Qualification]
[Professional title/post}

Specialist field:	Child and Adolescent Psychiatry
On behalf of :	[Mother's name]
On instructions of:	[——], Solicitors
Name of Subject:	Ann
Date of Birth of Subject	[——] (now aged 12 years)
Name of Subject:	Michael
Date of Birth of Subject:	[——] (now aged 10 years)
Name of Subject:	Susan
Date of Birth of Subject:	[——] (now aged 9 years)
Name of Subject:	William
Date of Birth of Subject:	[——] (now aged 3 years)
Legal Status of Subjects:	Residence order to [Father's name]
Subject Matter:	The children's contact with their mother

Court Reference Number:

Name and Address of Expert's Clinic/Hospital/Service
Telephone:
Fax:

Contents

Appendices

Appendix 1 –contains details of my experience and qualifications.

Appendix 2 –contains a list of the documents I have considered.

Appendix 3 –contains notes summarising the main points relevant to my report which are made in the documents read.

Appendix 4 –contains notes of my telephone conversation with Mrs P., family therapist, who was asked by the general practitioner to work with the family, and who provided a report for the court.

Appendix 5 –contains copies of the letters of instruction I have received.

Appendix 6 –contains a copy of my plan for the assessment.

Report of: [Expert's name]   Page no.
Specialist field: Child and Adolescent Psychiatry
On behalf of: [Name of Party]   **1.0 Introduction**

1.0   Introduction

1.1   Formal Details of Expert Witness

My full name is [Name/qualifications], [Job title/post].
(**Appendix 1** gives details of qualifications and experience.)

Area of specialisation: I qualified as a medical practitioner
in [Date]. I have specialised in psychiatry since ——, and in
child and adolescent psychiatry since——.

Source of instructions: I was requested to prepare this
report on behalf of the court by [——], solicitors, of
[Solicitors' address] in respect of private law proceedings
concerning contact between the children and their
mother, who also has applied for a residence order.

1.2   Synopsis

The four subjects of the proceedings have lived with their
father, [Father's name], since October 1990. Contact with
their mother, [Mother's name], was ordered by the court
in October 1990 and 1991. There have been difficulties
establishing contact, and the children have said that they
do not wish to see their mother. [Mother] would like
contact to be restored, and has made an application for a
residence order for all four children.

1.3   Instructions

The letters of instruction are attached as **Appendix 5**. I
have been asked to review the papers relating to the case,
and to give an opinion about the children's contact with
their mother.

1.4   Disclosure of Interests

(i) I have reviewed the documents provided, and have
identified a number of gaps in the information needed
to give a definitive opinion on the issues in question.

(ii) I have no connection with any of the parties, witnesses
or advisers involved in the case.

Report of: [Expert's name]   Page no.
Specialist field: Child and Adolescent Psychiatry
On behalf of: [Name of Party]   **2.0 Background**

2.0   The Background to the Dispute and the Issues

2.1   The Relevant Parties

[Mother's name] – mother of the children who are the subjects of the report.

[Father's name] – father of the children, and with whom the children reside.

2.2   The Assumed Facts

The children have become hostile to having contact with their mother.

2.3   The Issues to be Addressed

I have been asked to address the questions detailed in Section 4 below.

Report of: [Expert's name]   Page no.
Specialist field: Child and Adolescent Psychiatry
On behalf of: [Name of Party]   **3.0 Assessment**

3.0   The Psychiatric Assessment

This consisted only of appraisal of the documents submitted, as requested. I did not have leave to see the children or their parents.

The documents read are listed in **Appendix 2**.

The main points relevant to the questions at issue are listed in **Appendix 3**.

Summary of Appraisal of Documents

3.1   The children lived with [Mother's name] following the separation of their parents in 1989 and had regular contact with their father. In July 1990, [Father's name] failed to return the children to the care of their mother because of his concerns about [Mother's] care of the children. His allegations were not accepted by the court and the children were returned to [Mother] pending the final hearing in October 1990. At that time it was agreed by the mother and father that the children should live with [Father] and have regular contact with [Mother]. Since the children have been with [Father] regular contact has not been established. I have seen no evidence to suggest that [Father] has been active in encouraging and supporting the children to have contact with their mother. An allegation of sexual abuse by the mother's cousin was made by Ann in March 1991, and was the subject of a child protection investigation. No further action was taken.

3.2   Both parents are said to provide good care of the children. However, since Ann made the allegation of sexual abuse, [Father] has made a number of allegations that [Mother] is neglectful and abusive towards the children. In addition, allegations have been made by [Mother] that [Father] has been involved in sexual abuse with the children of his previous marriage, and that he has been emotionally abusive towards Ann, Michael, Susan and William. The allegations raise serious questions about the parenting

Report of: [Expert's name]   Page no.
Specialist field: Child and Adolescent Psychiatry
On behalf of: [Name of Party]   **3.0 Assessment**

abilities of both parents. The available documents do not make clear whether these allegations have been reported to the appropriate authorities, and if so, what the outcome was. The letter from Dr M. (general practitioner) about his examination of William's finger warts at the father's request [date of letter inserted] states that the damage to the warts is "consistent with a cigarette burn".

3.3   Concern has been expressed by officers of the [county] Social Services Department, the Court Welfare Officer and the court about the potentially harmful effect of parental acrimony on the children. Two years ago the children were described as beginning to show signs of emotional stress and physical illness related to times of contact with their mother, and as having attempted to avoid contact. They are reported as having spoken of their mother being neglectful and abusive in her treatment of them. They are also reported as having had a good relationship with their mother up to a year ago, and of stating that they wanted to live with her. [Mother] has stated that she thinks that [Father] is turning the children against her. [Father] states that the children simply do not want to see their mother.

Report of: [Expert's name]   Page no.
Specialist field: Child and Adolescent Psychiatry
On behalf of: [Name of Party]   **4.0 Conclusions**

4.0   Conclusions

4.1   General Conclusions

The emotional needs of the children and the reasons for their emotional difficulties, including their avoidance of contact with their mother, have not been fully assessed from a psychiatric point of view. The relationship of the children with their parents, and the ability of the parents to meet the children's needs have not been assessed taking full account of the allegations of abuse that have been made by [Father], the allegations of coercion that have been made by [Mother], and what could be done to overcome the acrimony between the parents. The terms of reference for the work carried out by Mrs P. and her colleagues, and which is described in her report of [Date], did not include a brief to explore these areas of concern. I have not seen the children or their parents personally, and have therefore not been able to make my own assessment of these issues. It is therefore difficult for me to provide definitive answers to the questions asked. The answers provided below must be taken as provisional, and will be in need of revision in the light of additional information.

4.2   Specific questions asked

4.2.1 What are the causes of the children's hostility to their mother?

From the information available to me, it is not clear whether the children are actually hostile to their mother, or are wishing to avoid contact with her. This would benefit from further assessment. The information currently available suggests four main possibilities:

(i) It is possible that the children have experienced abuse and neglect while in the care of their mother. Numerous allegations of abuse and neglect have been made by [Father] and the children since the time that the children have lived with him. It is not clear whether

Report of: [Expert's name]   Page no.
Specialist field: Child and Adolescent Psychiatry
On behalf of: [Name of Party]   **4.0 Conclusions**

these allegations have been reported to the appropriate authorities, and if so, whether they were substantiated. The allegations of sexual abuse of Ann by [Mother's] uncle have been substantiated. The other allegations do not appear to have been substantiated. There does not appear to have been any detailed formal assessment of the mother's parenting abilities since these allegations were made. Witness statements and the Court Welfare Officer's reports of 1990 and 1991 suggest that the mother's parenting is satisfactory. [Father's] allegations of poor parenting by the mother have not been supported by the Child Protection Conference or the court. Dr M.'s (GP) letter regarding William's warts is open to a number of interpretations and does not resolve questions about how the alleged injury was caused, and whether it was accidental or deliberate.

The written documents suggest a number of other possibilities which have not been fully investigated. These include the possibility that the allegations of abuse could have been malicious; could have arisen from misunderstanding; or could have resulted from lack of adequate communication between [Father] and [Mother].

(ii) [Father] fears that the children will experience abuse and neglect when they visit their mother, and it is possible that he has communicated these fears to the children. [Father] has repeatedly stated his fears that [Mother] is unable to provide adequate care for the children. He does not appear to have been able to discuss with [Mother] whether these fears have any basis in fact, nor has there been any discussion between the parents about practical steps that can be taken to reduce these fears. [Father] has stated that he thinks that it is in the children's interests to have contact with their mother, but is not on record as stating his reasons for this. His written evidence and Mrs P.'s assessment give no indication as to whether or not [Father] is aware of the importance of parental contact

Report of:	[Expert's name]	Page no.
Specialist field:	Child and Adolescent Psychiatry	
On behalf of:	[Name of Party]	**4.0 Conclusions**

for the children. Given his view that [Mother] is unable to provide for the children's needs, and that the children are at risk of abuse and neglect while with her, it is difficult to see how [Father] could believe that contact with their mother could be of benefit to the children. Given his beliefs, it would not have been easy for him to support the children having contact with their mother. There is nothing in the documents that I have seen to show that [Father] has in fact been able to provide encouragement and practical support of the kind that would enable the children to have contact with their mother. In these circumstances, and given the history of conflict between the parents and the current animosity between them, it is likely that the children feel very anxious about contact with their mother.

I am aware that my information may be incomplete, and that these impressions may therefore be inaccurate. This area would benefit from further assessment. It does not appear to have been included in the terms of reference for Mrs P.'s report.

(iii)   It is possible that the animosity between the parents could contribute to the children's hostility to contact with their mother. The assessments carried out to date do not address this issue directly. However, the evidence that is currently available suggests that it is very unlikely that the children are not aware of the animosity that exists between their parents. This awareness, combined with the repeated disruptions they have experienced, is likely to contribute to the children feeling caught in a conflict of loyalties and to be very anxious about further disruption. Symptoms of anxiety in children of this age are often expressed in terms of physical complaints and avoidant behaviour. The children are likely to want to avoid doing anything that would increase the risk of conflict and disruption. The Court Welfare Officer's report [date, page xx] states that the care provided by the children by both parents is good. However, since

Report of: [Expert's name]   Page no.
Specialist field: Child and Adolescent Psychiatry
On behalf of: [Name of Party]   **4.0 Conclusions**

the children are currently living with their father an easy way of avoiding further upset, disruption and conflict would be to avoid contact with their mother.

These possibilities would, in my view, benefit from further assessment.

(iv) It is possible that the children's hostility to contact with their mother could be caused by fear of their father, or a wish to please him. This possibility has not been assessed clinically, and would need to be looked at as part of a more detailed assessment of the children's relationship with their father than is currently available. The evidence now available suggests that [Father's] care of the children is good and that they have a good relationship with him. In these circumstances, it would be normal for the children to want to please their father. Their past experience of domestic violence and animosity between the parents (described in Document 1, page 4 – see **Appendix 2**), breakdown of the family and loss of contact with their mother are likely to make them wish to avoid displeasing him. Given their past experience, the children are likely to fear that there could be further parental conflict, violence or loss if contact occurs. The degree to which the children actually are affected in this way could be clarified by further assessment.

4.2.2   What is the likely reaction of Ann, Michael and Susan to being present when their mother collects William?

The evidence suggests that the children currently avoid being present on these occasions. The underlying reasons for this avoidance have not been fully assessed. However, it is clear that if there is an atmosphere of animosity between the parents, the children are likely to feel anxious about the possibility of parental conflict and to wish to avoid any contact with the mother. On the other hand, if there was less animosity between [Father] and [Mother], and if they were able to agree

Report of: [Expert's name]   Page no.
Specialist field: Child and Adolescent Psychiatry
On behalf of: [Name of Party]   4.0 **Conclusions**

that contact was in the children's best interests and to cooperate in relation to the arrangements, these meetings could provide an opportunity for the children to see their mother and re-establish contact.

4.2.3 What can be done to minimise the effects on the children of the animosity between the parents?

This important question has not been addressed as part of the assessments carried out to date, and was not part of the terms of reference of Mrs P.'s report. Considerable concern has been expressed about the possible harmful effects on the children of the animosity between [Father] and [Mother]. To date, this animosity has caused the children to experience domestic violence, the breakdown of the family, the loss of their home and the loss of contact with their mother and her extended family, and the experience of continuing parental conflict. All of these constitute serious risk factors for significant harm to the psychological health and well-being of the children. Given that the care of both parents is said to be good, the children are likely to benefit from continuing contact with both parents. However, at present the continuing animosity between the parents appears to make it very difficult to achieve. The children would benefit from a reduction in the animosity between their parents to the extent that they are able to consider the best interests of the children and cooperate in promoting these. In particular, the children would benefit if [Father] and [Mother] were able to cooperate over arrangements for contact with the non-custodial parent. The evidence currently available suggests that [Mother] and [Father] would be unlikely to be able to achieve this without considerable help, and that they have not, to date, been offered help of this kind.

4.2.4 What is the likely effect on the children of developing a negative attitude to their mother at a time when they are not having any contact with her?

Report of: [Expert's name]   Page no.
Specialist field: Child and Adolescent Psychiatry
On behalf of: [Name of Party]   4.0 Conclusions

The children's apparent hostility to contact with their mother and the allegations of bad parenting that they have made about her have resulted in contact with their mother effectively being lost. The effects of this on each of the children has not been fully assessed, and detailed material is therefore not yet available.

It is now well known that the loss of a parent in early childhood is an important risk factor for the future mental health of the child. The precise nature of the effects will depend on the nature of the relationship that has been lost, the developmental stage of the child and the degree to which the child's needs can be met following the loss. The effect of the loss of an abusive parent is likely to be complicated by the effects of the abuse experienced. The loss of a non-abusive parent is normally very traumatic, and can have long-lasting effects on the child's later mental health and emotional well-being. In the case of loss as a result of parental separation or divorce, the harmful effects can be minimised where the parents are able to set aside their personal differences and cooperate in providing for the child's best interests. In the case of young children, it is normally in the child's best interests to have frequent and regular contact with the non-residential parent.

4.2.5 Are the children of an age to be able to make informed decisions about contact with their mother? Would it benefit the children to re-establish contact with their mother?

The documents available suggest that contact has been progressively discontinued on the basis of the children's perceived hostility (by father) to contact with their mother. However, the children are much too young to be able to make informed decisions regarding their own best interests, especially in matters as important as this. Also, as mentioned above, there are a number of

Report of: [Expert's name]   Page no.
Specialist field: Child and Adolescent Psychiatry
On behalf of: [Name of Party]   **4.0 Conclusions**

possibilities as to why the children might wish to avoid contact, and these would benefit from further assessment.

The assessment carried out by Mrs P. was limited in scope, being based mainly on an agreement with [Father] to carry out therapeutic work with the children. A number of important areas were not included in the terms of reference of the work. In particular, no provision was made for exploration of the following areas: the role of parental animosity in the children's avoidance of contact with their mother; the parent–child relationship, including parental ability to identify the children's needs as separate from their own, and be able to respond appropriately; the reasons for the animosity between the parents and whether this could be set aside for the benefit of the children; whether they could be helped to discuss issues of concern and to cooperate in order to promote the children's best interests. The therapeutic help carried out by Mrs P. pre-dated the assessment requested by the court, and did not include any component of help for [Father] and [Mother] in how they might collaborate more effectively as parents.

The children are likely to benefit from a further assessment of these issues. The parents may benefit from being offered some help to resolve their difficulties. If the assessment concludes that the children's best interests would be served by having contact with both parents, consideration will need to be given as to what therapeutic help may need to be given in order to achieve this, and what type of legal support may be needed. If the assessment concludes that parental animosity is a major factor preventing the children's needs for parental contact from being met, questions may arise about which parent is likely to be able to meet the children's need for contact with the non-custodial parent most effectively. The risk of significant harm due to lack of contact may need to be weighed against the risk of significant harm due to the effects of parental conflict.

Report of: [Expert's name]   Page no.
Specialist field: Child and Adolescent Psychiatry
On behalf of: [Name of Party]   **4.0 Conclusions**

4.2.6 What can be done to help the children to reduce their hostile feelings towards their mother, and re-establish contact?

The possible reasons for the children's hostility to their mother have been discussed above. The help needed to reduce their hostility will depend on the underlying reasons for it. If the children have experienced abuse from their mother, then help may be needed to prevent this from happening again, and help her to provide more appropriate care. It might be beneficial to the children if [Father's] fears that the children may be abused by their mother were discussed, and attempts made to reassure him about the provisions that have been made to safeguard the children's safety. Reduction in parental animosity would help to reduce any anxieties that the children may have about conflict, violence and loss of parental love. Fears that the children may have of exacerbating the animosity between their parents would be helped by the opportunity to discuss these fears, and by the parents being able to demonstrate that they are willing to cooperate in the children's best interests.

4.2.7 What are the possible effects of change of residence on each of the children at this stage?

From the information available to me, it is not clear that a change of residence would be in the children's best interests. This would benefit from independent assessment. The effects of a change of residence would depend upon a number of factors. The nature of the change proposed, the ways in which the change would be likely to improve the chances of the children's needs being met, the wishes and feelings of the children, and the way in which these could be taken into account. More detailed information is required about the current psychological needs of the children, the degree to which their needs are currently thought to be met,

Report of: [Expert's name]   Page no.
Specialist field: Child and Adolescent Psychiatry
On behalf of: [Name of Party]   **4.0 Conclusions**

and the risks that might follow from disruption of their present placement.

4.3   Recommendations

I would respectfully recommend to the court that the children would benefit from a specialist assessment of their emotional needs by an independent expert.

I would further recommend a more detailed assessment of the abilities of the parents to meet the needs of the children and of what help they may need to set aside their personal differences in order to resolve their concerns about abuse of the children and to cooperate more effectively in providing for the best interests of the children. Some assessment of their ability to make use of the help available would also be useful.

Such an assessment is likely to require a number of meetings, and may need to be followed up with ongoing work. It would therefore probably be most conveniently undertaken by the local child psychiatric team.

I declare that this statement is true to the best of my knowledge information and belief and I understand that it may be placed before the court.

Signature _____

Name   _____ [Name/qualifications]

Date   _____

Mother kills father: report on an adolescent daughter

This report, written at the request of a 14-year-old girl's guardian ad litem, illustrates the complexity of cases involving intra-familial homicide. Although accepting the validity of the local authority care plan to attempt rehabilitation, the expert was doubtful about the likelihood of success unless there was intensive therapeutic input. This did not eventuate; the girl nevertheless returned to her mother, continued to abscond and the last news was that she was living rough, having reached her majority.

(HEADED PAPER)

(DATE)

Psychiatric Report

Re: CINDY BEER (d.o.b. — — — : now aged 14 years)

Case reference: (——)

Contents

I   Introduction

1   I was asked by the guardian ad litem's solicitors, Bloggs and Bloggs, to read the papers in this case and give a preliminary opinion about Cindy. Having read the papers I decided I would have to meet her and, with the court's permission, I travelled to see her at her secure unit on (date), when I also met her mother, her sister, Laura, her present keyworker (name), and her social worker (name). I was assisted by our psychology intern, Miss M.

My qualifications

2   (paragraph here)

Documents read

3   I have read the papers listed in the Appendix. I have been asked to deal with the following issues:

(a) The ascertainable wishes and feelings of Cindy, considered in the light of her age and understanding.

(b) Her physical, emotional and educational needs.

(c) The likely effect on her of any change in her circumstances.

(d) Her age, background and any characteristics of her which may be relevant.

(e) Any harm which she may have suffered or is at risk of suffering.

(f) How capable the mother and any other person in relation to whom I consider the question to be relevant, is of meeting her needs.

(g) The prospects of rehabilitation in full or in part and the timetables in respect thereof.

(h) Any other matter which I consider to be relevant and appropriate.

II   Brief history

4   Cindy, aged 14, is the elder of two sisters, both of whom were received into care by Wessex Local Authority after

the death of their putative father at their mother's hands, when Cindy was eight years old. Laura has now returned to her mother's care. Cindy had a large number of different foster placements in children's homes, her placements breaking down mainly because of repeated absconding. It is not clear when this began, but a list of abscondings prepared by her social worker indicated that between the ages of 11 and 13 Cindy had absconded no less than 40 times and had been picked up in most parts of the country. This may not be a complete list. Mention is made in the social profile, which is undated and unsigned, that Cindy began absconding when she was 11, shortly before her mother was granted a programme of home leave to visit her children.

5   On many of these occasions she was accompanied by her younger sister. There had been several petty thieving offences, although her behaviour generally when she was with her foster parents was considered to be good. As a result of the difficulty in ensuring Cindy's safety, a Secure Accommodation Order was made for three months when she was 13, and Cindy currently resides at a secure unit, where a further Secure Accommodation Order was made for six months.

6   Cindy's mother was found not guilty of murder but guilty of manslaughter due to provocation and received a seven-year sentence, but was released on parole when Cindy was 12 and a half. Both children were returned to their mother's care and while Laura settled well, Cindy became increasingly violent towards her mother and her sister and continued her pattern of frequent absconding. Following this she was accommodated by the local authority and placed in a children's home with educational facilities on the premises.

III   Psychiatric involvement

7   Cindy and her sister were referred to the consultant child and adolescent psychiatrist, at Wessex NHS Trust Hospital,

when Cindy was 10 years old. He kindly made his clinic's file on Cindy available to me with her permission. Cindy saw a psychiatric nurse for 18 months for weekly psychotherapy sessions. The work was interrupted by Cindy's repeated absconding and by her placement at the secure unit.

8   The papers were also read by Dr A., a consultant in child and adolescent psychiatry at South Hospital, who did not see the children. His report is a useful summary of the papers. He advised that on the face of it rehabilitation was not an appropriate aim for Cindy. I understand that there is a psychiatrist visiting the secure unit but I have not seen a report from him or her.

IV   Other assessment and therapeutic work

9   Various social workers have undertaken both assessments and counselling work with the children, including bereavement counselling while at the secure unit by Cindy's keyworker, Mrs J.

V   Interviews (date)

Cindy

10   I arrived at the secure unit at approximately 11.00. I had hoped to meet Cindy's mother first, but she was delayed because of fog. After a short orientation session with Cindy's key social worker I met Cindy, who was expecting me. She is an attractive pubertal young teenager who is articulate and forthcoming and gave a good account of herself. I explained to her that I had been asked by the court to help advise about her future care and placement. She told me she knew she was at the secure accommodation unit because she had run away so many times. She said that she began running away because her foster parents were talking badly about her

father and she could not bear it. After a while she thought she got into the habit of running away, especially when anyone mentioned anything about her Dad she would run. Altogether she has been in three foster homes, and she had returned briefly to the second family. She had also been in a children's home. She said she had mixed feelings about her mother the whole time. Cindy knew that her Dad was doing 'bad things' to her Mum that she did not like because her Mum had told her. She herself remembered how her Dad had shouted at her and about how they had thrown crockery at each other. Her Dad often used to send them to their rooms. She recalled that at one time her parents had decided to separate and she and her sister had wanted to stay with their Mum. They went to live with a friend of their Mum's, and their Mum went away and did not come back. She learnt that her Dad had been killed when she saw it on the television a few days later, but no one ever talked to her about it and she pretended she did not know. She was just told that her Mum was in prison and that her Dad was dead, and to this day her Mum has not told Cindy the details of the killing. When she asks about it, she is told it is as it was reported in the papers which she has read.

11 Recently, since Cindy has been working with Mrs J., she has been asking her Mum more, and her mother has been talking to her about what happened and about the fear she had that their Dad would kill her, Cindy and Laura.

12 I asked Cindy to tell me about her father. She described him as having fair hair, being tall and wearing horrible shirts. He would get very angry with them at times. He was quite scary, especially when they woke him up. Cindy thought that her Grandma, Dad's mother, was scared of her father too and that he had stopped Grandma from seeing them. The good things about him were that on holidays he would take her sister and her to a huge shopping centre and buy them nice things and he used to take them out a lot. She said that she thought the good memories of him balanced out the bad ones. I asked her

---

Psychiatric report: Cindy BEER
Dr (Psychiatrist's name)

Case reference: (——)
(Date)

how she would have liked things to have been different, and she said that she would have made her father's temper better so that he would have treated her mother better and then he would be alive.

13   Cindy told me that her mother had told her that at the time she saw killing Cindy's father as the only way of preventing him from harming them, and that she now realises it was wrong and that there would have been other solutions. Cindy remembers her mother was very sad and became thinner around the time of her Dad's death. At first she felt scared of her Mum but she is less worried now and she believes that her mother would now go and talk to someone if she had worries rather than acting as she did against her father. Cindy told me that she used to worry that it might have been something she said on that day that caused her Mum to act as she did but she now does not believe that she was at fault, although Grandma had placed the blame on the girls.

14   We talked about her running away and she thought that she had now kicked the habit. She denied having any sexual experiences while she was away, but admitted that she had tried cannabis. She recalled running away when she was living with her mother because they were always fighting.

15   Cindy values the sessions that she has regularly with her social worker, Mrs J. She showed me some of the work she had done with her, which was learning a little about grief and how loss affects people. She also recalled the work that she had done with Mrs W. in Wessex.

16   Cindy told me that she ate and slept well, and that she had made friends with the other four girls in her secure unit. She said that she was hoping to move to the open unit there and eventually to return home to her mother. She saw all this as taking many months. Currently she is having education on the premises and she believes she is doing well. She enjoys her schooling. We talked a bit about her father and the fact that he had had epilepsy

and whether that might account for his violence. She would like to talk to people who knew her father before the epilepsy to find out what he was like. She is aware that she has something of her father in her and thinks that this is why she did not get on with her mother when she went home.

Cindy's mother

17   Cindy's mother then arrived with Laura and the social worker. I saw the mother alone. She told me how her husband would lie in bed and scream and shout at her. It was when he would lock the children in their room for minor naughty behaviour, such as taking a biscuit, that she decided that she would kill him. She had tried to leave him in the past but he always found her. At one point he made her take his pills, holding a knife to her throat saying he wanted her to have to get her stomach pumped out. She saw him as very sadistic. Cindy's mother said she knew nothing of the pornographic pictures her husband had had taken of Cindy. It was Cindy herself who told her mother about them. The father's violence really started after Cindy was born. The mother told Cindy's maternal grandmother how unhappy she was, but the grandmother encouraged her to stay with him. She often told her husband that she hated him but she did not know how to get free of him. She pointed out that his ex-wife had had to move abroad to get rid of him.

18   I asked Cindy's mother what help she had had for herself. She said that she had had no counselling in prison, although she had had some education, was hoping to study, and she has ambitions. She was particularly upset that she had never seen anyone from the Wessex Hospital when staff were offering treatment to her children, and she appreciated the work that was being done by Mrs J., but in reply to my question she said that there had been no family therapy sessions as yet. I discussed with her the possibility of Cindy meeting some of her father's family so that she could learn more about her father when he

was younger and before he had epilepsy. She said she would not object to this but she did not know how easy it would be to arrange. She believes she has a much stronger relationship with Cindy now. She said she had no problems with Laura, who recalled only bad memories about father.

Meeting with social workers

19   I then met with Cindy's current social worker, her keyworker and the head of the secure accommodation unit. I was told that Cindy was living with four other girls in a small house, which I was shown, which has nine staff, and in addition, teaching staff who come in. Cindy is not posing any management problems but is described as being very wrapped up in herself. She is the youngest there but there are other girls near her own age. Three of the girls in the unit are there for their own protection and one is there for an offence, so the majority of the girls are in a situation very similar to Cindy's. When she first came into the unit she had some difficulty in falling asleep and had some early morning wakening but she is now sleeping normally. At first she ate obsessively and gained about 10 pounds. Now she is back to her normal weight and she enjoys food normally. She has good social relationships with the group and although she is the youngest she is something of a leader. There have been no attempts at absconding, even though she has had opportunities when they have been on outings.

20   Cindy's current social worker has only been with Cindy for the past six months. Cindy is being held under a Secure Accommodation Order. I asked him about the involvement of his department prior to the killing. There was a report when Cindy was four that the children were not being supervised properly, which they investigated. The files were then closed until she was nine when they were asked in after the killing. I asked about the complaints that Cindy made about her foster parents.

He told me that the foster mother had admitted smacking the girls on their legs but had reported it to the department and their impression of the foster parents, who they have known for many years, is good.

21   I asked whether there had been any therapeutic work done with Laura and her mother since Laura had returned home but I understood that there had not been any. The only work that had been done as a family was during the assessment process. The reports on Laura at school have been good.

22   Mrs J. talked about the bereavement counselling that she had been doing with Cindy. She has a very warm relationship with her and is very impressed by Cindy, whom she sees as honest and troubled. Her intention is to work at a slow pace consistent with Cindy's wish to take things slowly. She hopes that Cindy will be able to move to the open unit in a month or two, and the time-scale that Cindy and the social worker are aiming at is to return Cindy to her mother's care in about six months' time. They anticipate that they will be carrying out some joint family work before then and that there will be periods at home on trial. I asked about the pornographic photographs and was told that the police had never found any evidence, and Cindy could not be specific about who had taken them so the matter was dropped. I asked about Cindy's attitude to sexuality and whether there had been any abnormal sexual behaviour at the secure unit. Apart from a certain crudity about sexual matters there have been no concerns about her, although the fact that she absconded so many times and was found with older girls far from home made people worried about her.

Laura

23   I saw Laura with Cindy, her mother and the social workers for a final meeting before I left. Laura is a lively 11-year-old who is able to give a good account of herself, but I felt there was a lot of denial of her earlier experiences.

I asked her who she would go to if she had a problem and she said she did not know. I got the impression that she would not necessarily go to her mother and she felt she did not know the social worker very well. She knew that the nurse whom she had seen at Wessex Hospital had left. When I had been talking to her mother she and Cindy had gone off together very happily and had shared things in an intimate way.

VI   Summary and opinion

24   Cindy is the elder of two girls. When she was nine her mother was arrested for her part in the death of their father. The mother was released from prison two years ago. The bundle of papers that I have seen relating to the mother's trial indicates that her husband was a very abusive husband and father. His previous wife's evidence is important in this regard. It is possible that his abusive behaviour was related to his operation for epilepsy which he had at the age of 20. There is no evidence about his previous personality; I would think it was important to try to get evidence of what he was like before his epilepsy, for Cindy's and Laura's sake. Although Cindy has some good memories of her father, if and when she returns to her mother's care it will be difficult for her mother to maintain those good memories and she needs to have evidence from another source. For that reason I recommend that her keyworker tries to trace the paternal relatives and gets an account of his earlier personality. This is particularly important as the mother sees Cindy as very like her father, and both she and Cindy are likely to interpret any behavioural problems as evidence that she is developing like her father. It may be that it will be found that the epilepsy is a 'red herring', and that the father's early behaviour was consistent with his later behaviour. That will call for a different approach to helping Cindy to come to terms with that part of her which is like her father.

Psychiatric report: Cindy BEER   Case reference: (——)
Dr (Psychiatrist's name)   (Date)

25   In my opinion the evidence from the notes that I have read of her therapist is that Cindy is frightened of 'catching manslaughteritis'. She has been able to recall a lot of unhappy memories about her father. I believe that it was the low esteem in which she held herself as a result of these recollections and fears that led to her persistent absconding. She was finding it difficult to face the pain from the insights she was gaining from the therapeutic work at the hospital and from the confrontations with her mother. It is important to note that she began to abscond not long after she started therapy and this coincided with her mother's release for home leave. I think it is true that it then became a habit and she took flight any time anyone mentioned anything painful. She has some insight into this herself and now that she no longer can take flight she is beginning to tackle some of these issues.

26   She has a good relationship with Mrs J., the social worker at the secure unit, who sees herself as offering bereavement counselling. Cindy will need skilled and prolonged psychotherapy in order to deal with the problems she has, and the difficulty is that her placement in the secure unit prevented her from commencing psychotherapy with a trained psychotherapist, Dr V. at Wessex Hospital. Mrs J. is aware that she is not able to offer the level of skill and expertise necessary for this girl and I am not sure if there is anyone else who would have the time or skill necessary while she is at the secure unit. One possibility would be Dr X., who is a psychotherapist based near the secure unit, and I would recommend that Mrs J. discusses this case with him and perhaps receives some supervision from him or one of his colleagues which would support her and enhance her work. It would be important to make sure that Dr V. has a vacancy to take Cindy on when she returns eventually to her mother.

27   I have some serious concerns about whether Cindy and indeed Laura, when she reaches adolescence, will find it easy to stay with their mother. Cindy certainly has

recollections of being neglected by her mother. She describes the way that her parents went out, pretending to leave them with babysitters when there were in fact no babysitters present. She recalled more affection from her father than her mother and this may well be because her mother was terrorised by her husband (she described how he insisted that she went out leaving the children as babies and nailing lids on their cots to prevent them from getting out). In my experience it is very difficult for children to understand how such terror can prevent a parent from protecting them and I believe that unless skilled and intensive work is done with Cindy, Laura and their mother together in family therapy, the home situation will not hold.

28   In a series of 22 children we have seen, where the mother has killed the father, many of the killings were done after years of abuse of the mother by the father (see Harris-Hendriks *et al* (1993) for an overview of interparental homicide). However, the problem for the children when they returned to the care of the mother, as they invariably did, there being much sympathy for the mother because of the evidence that is produced of her having been emotionally and physically battered often over a long period of time by the man she killed, is that they are unable to understand that the risk of mother killing again is slight. In our study we found that the predominant feeling is one of fear that if they should misbehave the same fate will be meted out to them as to their father. In the cases where the children have been returned to the care of the parent who has killed they do not do well.

29   In adolescence, in particular, they tend to rebel against the discipline and control exerted by the parent and challenge his or her moral right to control them on the grounds that because they have offended they are not able to exert authority. I think that it would be essential for there to be ongoing support and oversight of these children until they reach their majority.

30   If there is a Care Order in effect for Cindy, in addition to the Secure Accommodation Order, I would recommend that this be continued and that when Cindy does return home next summer there is close monitoring by social services. If Cindy resumes her absconding this should be taken as an indication that it is not possible to rehabilitate her with her mother. If there is no Care Order, one should be applied for before Cindy is released from the unit.

31   In my opinion the grounds for establishing that Cindy has been significantly harmed, and would be at risk of further harm without an Order, are present.

VII   Conclusions

Cindy's wishes and feelings

32   Cindy was returned to her mother's care in spite of contraindications to this being her wish, present in her consistent statements. The placement broke down quickly and she became habituated to absconding as a way of avoiding painful feelings and experiences. In the five months she has been in a secure unit she has begun to address some of these painful issues with her keyworker, with whom she has a good relationship. Cindy's wish at the moment is to work towards returning home next year. She is aware of the amount of work that needs to be done with her mother before this will be possible.

Her physical, emotional and educational needs

Her physical needs

33   Cindy has never had a full paediatric examination that includes an inspection of her genitalia. Although permission from Cindy would be needed for this to be done, in my opinion it is important that it is established that she has not had any sexual relationships. If she has, it would be important to ascertain her HIV status and also to counsel her with regard to contraception. Her physical needs for protection, shelter and nourishment are of course being

adequately met at present. I have no reason to believe that they would not be if she returned to her mother's care, unless she began absconding again.

Her emotional needs

34   She is at present partially alienated from her only parent, her mother, and from other members of her family. She requires psychotherapeutic treatment to help her come to terms with her family history including that of her father, her father's death, her mother's part in this and her genetic inheritance.

Her educational needs

35   Cindy appears to be a bright girl and her educational needs are probably not being fully met by attendance at the school unit on the premises. When she moves to the open unit I recommend that she attends a mainstream school in the locality.

Likely effect on her of any change in her circumstances

36   I think she is being well cared for physically and emotionally at present. However, she may well escalate her disturbed behaviour if attempts are made to return her home prematurely. There is a very real risk that even when she returns home in due course she will not be able to cope with living with her mother unless there is some intensive and skilled therapeutic work done with the family together.

Her age, background and characteristics which may be relevant

37   Cindy is pubertal. She has had many adverse experiences including physical and emotional abuse, possible sexual abuse, bereavement, a poor relationship with her mother, low self-esteem and a violent inheritance. The pattern of her behaviour indicates that her prognosis is not good and she is likely to have a delinquent career unless she receives adequate help.

Psychiatric report: Cindy BEER   Case reference: (——)
Dr (Psychiatrist's name)   (Date)

Any harm which she may have suffered or is at risk of suffering

38   Cindy and Laura were significantly harmed by the death of
their father at their mother's hands. They continued to
suffer significant harm during the periods their mother was
imprisoned because of their frequent changes of placement
and the frequent absconding. Cindy (and perhaps Laura
too) is at risk of suffering further significant harm if she
should be returned prematurely to her mother's care
without sufficient therapeutic work having been done.

Capability of the mother to meet her needs

39   Social services is not considering placement with any
other permanent carer than mother and I think on
balance that it is reasonable to try once again to rehabilitate
Cindy to her mother. I have considerable reservations
about whether this will be successful.

(a) Because the mother was abused she was unable to
stand against the children's father and allowed them
to be seriously at risk as infants and children because
they were left alone.

(b) She failed to protect them from their father's physical
and emotional abuse.

(c) She has not been offered, nor has she sought, any
therapy.

40   On the other hand she has accepted full responsibility for
what she did, apologised to the children and has consistently
cooperated with social services and the secure unit. Laura
has returned to her care without difficulty (although it must
be pointed out that Laura has not yet reached adolescence
when I expect the problems to begin). Cindy is no longer
being subjected to abuse or denigration and her mother's
self-esteem is now much higher than it was at the time she
and her husband were caring for their children.

41   If the mother was to accept therapy, where should it be
sought? I recommend that local services are consulted
about this. It may be that there are resources within
Wessex Hospital that could be offered.

Psychiatric report: Cindy BEER   Case reference: (——)
Dr (Psychiatrist's name)   (Date)

Prospects of rehabilitation and the timetable

42   In order for rehabilitation to have the maximum chance of success, in my opinion the following would be necessary:

   (a) Therapy for mother.
   (b) Individual psychotherapy for Cindy.
   (c) Family therapy sessions.
   (d) Increasing periods of trial placement at home.
   (e) Continued therapy after return home.
   (f) Termination of rehabilitation if absconding resumes or other symptoms occur which persist.
   (g) A properly agreed timetable with agreed termination criteria. I would be happy to advise on this if requested.
   (h) Any other matters.

Therapy

43   I refer to this in several places above. Dr X. should be consulted and Mrs J. may like to request supervision from his department or work with his department jointly, particularly in relation to work with the whole family. A therapist should be identified for the mother, providing she wishes it. Therapy will need to continue after Cindy's return home and Dr V.'s offer needs to be renegotiated.

Contact with the paternal family

44   The social services should seek out the paternal relatives to help Cindy to build up a picture of her father from childhood and certainly from before the onset of his epilepsy.

VIII Recommendations

45   (a) Cindy and her sister are entitled to criminal injury compensation and application should be made on their behalf by the local authority, if this has not already been done.

   (b) Cindy's placement is satisfactory. She is benefiting from it and it should be continued in order to enable her to be contained and continue therapy. She should be moved to the open unit as soon as possible and she should receive her education from an outside mainstream secondary school.

   (c) The therapeutic recommendations outlined above should be initiated.

   (d) Rehabilitation to the mother with the provisos outlined above should be given a trial with appropriate safeguards.

   (e) Any resumption of the absconding if she is returned home should be treated as evidence that the rehabilitation has failed.

   (f) She should be subject to a Care Order. I anticipate the Secure Accommodation Order can be allowed to lapse after six months.

   (g) I would be happy to remain available for consultation as appropriate.

I declare that this statement is true to the best of my knowledge information and belief and I understand that it may be placed before the court.

(name and qualifications)
Consultant Child and Adolescent Psychiatrist

Reference

Harris-Hendriks, J., Black, M. & Kaplan, T. (1993) *When Father Kills Mother: Guiding Children Through Trauma and Grief*. London: Routledge.

NB The original of this report and that which follows were laid out according to the guidelines in Chapter 3 but have been abbreviated to conserve space.

Psychiatric report: Cindy BEER   Case reference: (——)
Dr (Psychiatrist's name)   (Date)

Munchausen's syndrome by proxy: report on a three-year-old with developmental delay

This report contains a detailed account of the history of three children of a single parent where a diagnosis of Munchausen's syndrome by proxy is arrived at. Although the older brother is not the subject of the care proceedings, the expert draws attention to the need for him to be assessed given a similar history of near drowning and frequent presentation to doctors. The possibility that the 'cot death' of their brother might have been caused by smothering is not administrated, although, reading between the lines, it is clearly in the author's mind. The outcome of the case was that John was in due course adopted and did well. Peter was referred over a year later! He too was taken into care and placed in long-term foster care with regular contact with his mother. The latter never acknowledged that she had harmed the children and refused any help.

(HEADED PAPER)

(DATE)

Psychiatric Report

Re: JOHN JONES (d.o.b. — — — : now aged three years)

Case reference: (——)

Contents

I   Introduction

II   Background

III   Psychiatric interviews

Foster carer
Mother with the children
John and Peter alone with child psychotherapist
Mother with social worker

IV   Summary and opinion

Outline of Munchausen's syndrome by proxy
Responses to specific questions for consideration

V   Summary of recommendations

References
Appendix   List of documentation

I   Introduction

1   (Name(s) of author(s))

2   (Qualifications and experience)

3   We were asked to see this boy and his mother as a joint commission by the solicitors to Sunsetshire County Council (local authority solicitors), the solicitors to the mother (M.'s solicitors) and the solicitors to the guardian ad litem (guardian's solicitors) in a letter from (local authority solicitors), dated (——), in relation to care proceedings. We had letters from all three solicitors asking specific questions which I will deal with in section IV, Summary and opinion, of this report.

4   John, his mother and brother, Peter aged 10 and a half, his social worker, (social worker's name), and John's foster carer, (foster carer's name), were seen here on (date) by the (Clinic's name) team, comprising (name), senior family therapist, (name), senior child psychotherapist and myself.

Documents read

5   I have read the documents listed in the Appendix.

II   Background

6   John is the third child born to his mother – all by different fathers. John's father is alleged to be the mother's brother-in-law. The mother's first child, David, was born when she was not quite 18 and had been rejected by her family, and died at the age of 10 months of cot death. Peter currently lives with his mother and John is subject to an Interim Care Order made six months ago. He lives with a foster carer and has contact with his mother regularly.

7   The statement of Dr W., locum consultant paediatrician at Sunsetshire Hospital, dated (date) outlines John's medical history, which includes five admissions in the

first year of life, one in the second year and three in the third year to the date of his reception into care. The latter came about as his mother refused to take him home after the last admission, insisting that he was ill and should have a laparotomy or laparoscopy. Many of the previous admissions were on his mother's request when symptoms had been reported by her which were never observed by medical or nursing staff (these included screaming attacks, difficulty in swallowing, coughing and choking, asthma, allergies, lethargy, deafness, skin rash, tonsillitis, diarrhoea, fits, abdominal pain and threadworms). Two admissions resulted from incidents in which he had not been properly supervised (a near-drowning in the bath when left alone, and the ingestion of largactil tablets). In addition, John has had a few accidents. At one year of age he was seen in casualty when he fell downstairs and bruised his forehead, and at two years he crushed his left hand in a door. He was X-rayed because of a bony protuberance on his skull which worried his mother.

8   John's general practitioner records show 20 attendances in the first year, 17 in the second and 20 in the first seven months of his third year. There had been long-standing concerns about the mother's insistence on treatment for John, which medical staff did not think was justified, such as requests for tonsillectomy and for diets. She placed him on a dairy-free diet herself, and also on a gluten-free diet, suggesting that the dietician had placed him on it. This was denied by the latter, who said it was at the mother's suggestion. John's mother told her social worker that John was suffering from coeliac disease and asthma, which was not true.

9   John's development is delayed. He has a small head circumference (microcephaly) and delayed speech development. He has been seen by a large number of specialists mainly because of his mother's concerns about his health, but also because of some genuine problems, although these are not serious ones. He was investigated because of a heart murmur which is not significant or

harmful, he was to be circumcised because of phimosis, which improved before the operation, and there is a curious suggestion that he had some lumps on his penis.

10 The CONI records (special records kept by the mother recording symptoms in children born subsequent to a cot death) indicate the mother's concerns about John's chest and bowels in particular. They do not mention several of his admissions.

11 The health visitor's records indicate that the mother was a heavy smoker and did not modify her smoking habits even though advised to do so. She was in constant conflict with neighbours who made many calls to social services to complain of her treatment of the children. It is noted that the mother's handling of John is very negative – "constantly shouting and stopping him doing things" (health visitor records).

12 His relationship with his mother has been observed to be abnormal. He is unhappy if she approaches him, does not initiate contact with her and is indifferent to her departure.

13 His mother's health records and his brother Peter's show similar features to John's. On Peter's general practitioner records he was seen 19 times in his first year, 25 in his second and an average of 15 times a year thereafter to the present day. He has also nearly drowned on no less than three occasions (one 10 years ago and two the following year), has had innumerable hospital admissions, several apnoeic episodes in infancy and frequent accidents. He had difficulty in breathing after a caesarean delivery and had an apnoea alarm. He was on the 'at risk' register for a time and there were concerns about his failure to thrive and his mother's impatient and rough handling of him. Six years ago there is a record of a non-accidental injury inflicted by his mother, causing bruising to Peter's face and bleeding to his eye. He was admitted to hospital but no further action was taken. Four years ago his mother threatened to kill him.

Psychiatric report: John JONES   Case reference: (——)
Dr (Psychiatrist's name)   (Date)

14   The health visitor's record of John mentions that after the latter was placed with a foster carer, his mother complained of Peter's behaviour: "beating me up" and being disobedient. She expressed concern that he might be at risk sexually because he had a girlfriend.

15   The mother's medical records extend back to her childhood. She was a sickly child with recurrent ear infections, tonsillitis and many accidents. She was seen at the surgery as many times in her childhood as Peter has been. As an adult she has been castigated for her numerous out-of-hours calls to the general practitioner and has changed general practitioners several times. She has been accident prone in adult life too. There are many references to the mother's anger and dissatisfaction with her medical advisors.

16   I have not seen the medical records of David but the social work records indicate that he was admitted to hospital at a few weeks of age because of failure to thrive and was placed with foster carers at his mother's request at three months for a few weeks. It was noted that mother had a "rather rough and aggressive attitude" to the baby and there were concerns about her being able to cope. He was readmitted when he was five months because of screaming fits, which were not observed on the ward and there were concerns about the mother's handling of the baby. He failed to thrive for a time. His final illness was diagnosed post-mortem as acute bronchitis and cot death.

III   Psychiatric interviews on (date)

17   The children's mother, Peter and John were seen with their social worker (social worker's name) and John's foster carer (foster carer's name) at the (hospital's name). (Foster carer's name) was interviewed by our senior family therapist while the family were seen by our senior child psychotherapist and myself. She then saw the children alone, while I interviewed the mother alone.

Finally, the mother was left alone with both children while we observed the session through a one-way screen.

(Foster carer's name), foster carer

18   (Foster carer's name) lives with her husband and two children aged nine and 11. The couple have been foster carers for five years and have fostered special needs children before. They have had John's care for six months. She told us that at first John had a false smile all the time, as if he needed to reassure them, but it is now more appropriately used and he differentiates between strangers and those he knows. He was not very steady on his feet and does not seem aware of danger. His speech was very limited; he still has great difficulty in articulation although he understands more (but his understanding too is quite delayed). He is also quite negative about speaking. He likes routine and can be rather obsessional, for example he will not eat before he has his bib on. When he first came he could not dress himself but he is better at it now. He likes to be independent and is fairly good with his hands. He is able to untie shoelaces from a knot, can drink out of a cup and eat with a spoon. He is still in nappies. It does not bother him if he is wet and dirty. He does not have any idea of using a pot or toilet. He sleeps very well at night. His health has been good, apart from a couple of colds which he recovered from quickly.

19   Within a fortnight (foster care's name) had him on a normal diet (from a dairy-free, gluten-free one) with no problems at all. He attends a play group four mornings a week. He is reasonably sociable, is content to play on his own but he needs to be told to play otherwise he just follows her around. He is confident with strangers although he prefers men to women. He gets on well with her children. There have been no tantrums and he seems very placid. He goes happily to contact and comes back happily.

20   He likes to initiate contact for a cuddle. He goes stiff if anyone approaches him. He kisses everyone goodnight.

If he knocks into something or hurts himself, he crys but does not seek comfort. He is active in showing what he wants and anticipates – for example getting a towel for (foster carer's name) to dry his hands.

21 (Foster carer's name) had not observed him with his mother until today when they travelled together. He rejected all his mother's frequent overtures, pushing her away and saying "back, back". He refused to get into his pushchair when his mother asked him to.

Mother with the children

22 The social worker joined us for the early part of the meeting only.

23 Peter is a well grown sturdy boy who had a rash around his mouth at the time of the interview. He hovered near his mother, rather anxious and fidgety, making little use of the toys and refusing to draw. By contrast, John, an attractive toddler whose head (although small by measurement) appears normal, made a beeline for the toys and the small sink and enjoyed fairly constructive play throughout the session, with little reference to his mother. He was willing to, in fact eager to, relate to our child psychotherapist and myself, and although we heard little speech, he responded to our comments, brought things to show us and followed our suggestions. He also referred very little to his brother. When (foster carer's name) left the room, he appeared to be unperturbed.

24 We started by asking if the mother understood the purpose of the meeting. She said she did, so we invited her to explain it to the children. She immediately said "They think I've got Munchausen by proxy". We asked Peter if he understood that, and his mother said, "I think it is about being accused of child abuse – people seem to think I have been accused of making children have operations – I didn't demand it, I wanted to know why he was having all the symptoms – I didn't understand how a child could be constipated and still use his bowels. His

stools have been loose ever since he was born". I asked where the laparoscopy came in and his mother said that John's stomach was swollen and in view of the fact that she had lost a child as a result of a doctor's actions she wanted to find out if there was anything wrong. The mother denied she had asked for a laparoscopy or a laparotomy. She used a lot of medical jargon.

25   We explored with Peter his understanding of what his mother had said to him, and as it was obviously confusing for him we tried to reassure him.

26   His mother was asked about the idea of coeliac disease. She said she was constantly being told it was toddler's diarrhoea. "I took it into my own hands. Maybe I shouldn't have. I put him on a gluten-free diet, with the help of the dietician." She said that she was not worried about the heart murmur although she did not seem to have taken in that it was not pathological.

27   We asked about Peter's rash. This seemed to be caused by his constantly licking his lips and the area round them. His mother said that he had cream to put on them but that he did not use it, "He's 10 years old and I can't be behind him all the time". We asked if she could put it on and she said she kept telling him to do it, "As far as he's concerned, going out with friends is more important than caring for his lips." This was said very angrily.

28   We asked about Peter's illnesses. The mother gave a long list of asthma, chicken pox and tonsillitis until a tonsillectomy at seven years. Peter mentioned a fractured ankle. When we asked his mother about her childhood illness, Peter interrupted to say he had been in hospital 600 times and modified it to 15–16. Peter's mother denied this and there ensued an argument between them. His mother mentioned that he had been in once with concussion, once with tonsils and once with glasses. I asked Peter to show us how well he could read with his glasses, but although apparently concentrating on the book, he kept an ear open for the adult conversation.

His reading was not very fluent but he comprehended satisfactorily. Peter said his teacher forgot to remind him to wear his glasses. (He was not wearing them today.) The mother said both children were independent.

29 Discussing David, the baby who died, the mother saw it as the doctor's fault as he refused to come out when she called him. She had not realised he was so ill and her parents had thrown her out when she was pregnant so she could not get help from them, although she asked, or David's father, who was not there. As she was telling this story, Peter tried to interrupt and divert her, and answered for her, clearly trying to protect his mother and prevent her from being upset. He acknowledged this when we suggested that was what was happening. We asked him what would happen if he did not protect his mother, "She'd most probably tell you a load of lies, no not lies, but lots of other stories". At this point, for the first time he went to play with John. He said, in reply to a question directed to mother, "Uncle (name) is John's father". Peter tried to take some bricks from his brother, who started to cry. The children's mother did nothing, so we asked Peter to stop and got them to share. John was very amenable to giving some to his brother, saying "Dere", and was praised for doing so by us. The children played together for a short time. Peter kept an alert ear on the adult conversation, yet again answering for his mother when he felt she was getting agitated.

30 The children's mother told us a little about her own background. We asked if she had happy memories and she said she could not recall her parents ever sitting down with her. She was the sixth of seven children – her father was in the army and then worked on buses. She denied having significant health problems as a child and talked about her sister's current pregnancy with some resentment as her mother concentrated on her sister. Her father had died recently.

31 At this point the mother started to pay attention for the first time to John, perhaps to divert us from discussing

her childhood further. John was playing at the sink and she went to him. He began to scream and made movements with his hands to push her away and his mother immediately moved away. He settled down to play again and stopped screaming. His mother said he always screams when she moves near him. She went on to talk about a fall she had six years ago when she fractured her thumb, since which time she has problems with it. She is waiting for an admission to hospital.

32   We asked if there was any doctor she trusted and she said her current general practitioner. We heard about other doctors who had taken her off their list. We asked if she took the children's temperature when she thought they were febrile, but she said she only felt their head. She expressed anger with the children for being the way they were, "I didn't make them that way".

John and Peter alone with child psychotherapist

33   I took the children's mother into another room. Neither child protested at her leaving and seemed happy to be alone with the child psychotherapist. The mother did not prepare them for her departure but the child psychotherapist explained afterwards where she had gone and that she would be back soon. Neither child seemed concerned. In reply to questions about why they had come, Peter said that they had accused their Mum of saying they were ill when they were not. That was a "load of rubbish – its not true". Asked about hospital visits, "I've been in so many times its unbelievable", and he went on to describe some of the hospital visits. John then claimed the child psychotherapist's attention, by wiping his hands and asking for "bin-bin". When she approached him he shouted at her to go back. Peter said rather sadly, "It's taken me two and a half years to get used to John, and now if he gets back I suppose it will take me another two and a half years". The child psychotherapist queried this and he said he was used to being with his Mum by himself, "I

was used to all the care and attention". He thought he still had more attention than John, and certainly claimed more from the child psychotherapist. He said he tried to help his Mum with John, who was clumsy and it was very hard. He helped with bedtime and bathtime: "I find it really hard since he's gone to foster care". The child psychotherapist empathised with him and he went on to talk about how he could not leave his Mum alone as she needed him and he worried about her being ill so much. He did not understand why John went away and he was worried the same would happen to him. "Am I going to be taken into care?" he asked. "I'd find it hard to leave my Mum." The child psychotherapist asked him why he thought he might be taken into care, and he avoided her gaze, concentrating on the bricks, saying he only under-stood what Mummy told him. He thought the doctors were wrong, and sighed a lot, saying several times that he was finding it hard (meaning his life). The child psychotherapist asked if he remembered a time with his Mum when he had no worries. Peter pulled his arms into his sweatshirt and said that his Mum had always been difficult but strong. The child psychotherapist tried to explore this and asked if his Mum had said she was strong. He did not reply but looked at her and said again that he missed John.

34   During this time, John was playing with bricks and seemed happy in his own play. He was reasonably constructive, but resistant to anyone interfering. He took little notice of the above exchange and there was little spontaneous speech.

Mother alone

35   I asked the children's mother about her own childhood, having learned from the social worker about the mother's statement that she had been sexually abused by two of her brothers in childhood. When I expressed sympathy for her situation she replied that it would have been different if her family had helped her. Her older brothers sexually abused her from the age of six or seven. "They

were the only ones showing me love – I was grateful someone was noticing me. One would watch while the other one did it." She never told her mother. "I learned to live with it." One brother later became a transsexual. "It upset me. When someone has been sexually abusing you and then you discover he is a transsexual...". She said that he was now married and had had a child who died with congenital abnormalities within hours of birth.

36   The mother's mother lost both parents when she was seven and was brought up in an orphanage. John and Peter's mother thought this accounted for her coldness.

37   Asked if she had ever had any treatment from a psychiatrist, she mentioned that she had seen a community psychiatric nurse, at the request of her health visitor, and was given a clean bill of health.

Mother with social worker

38   We were joined by the child psychotherapist. I told the children's mother that I would not be able to give an opinion until I had read all the papers. The child psychotherapist wondered if the mother would be prepared to have some therapy. The child psychotherapist explained that therapy was a confidential relationship with someone trained and experienced in helping to understand how past experiences influence present behaviour, and that the therapist worked with their client to find ways of changing attitudes, feelings and behaviour. The mother said she did not want therapy but she would go through with it if it meant she could get John back. The child psychotherapist went on to say it would be someone for her who might help with her worries. The mother said she had no worries at home. She felt she had done a good job with Peter and only accepted that the diet was the one thing she had done wrong with John. John's mother said, "If I say I don't want to have therapy, does it mean I haven't a chance to get John back? If it is recommended, I'll take it".

Psychiatric report: John JONES   Case reference: (——)
Dr (Psychiatrist's name)   (Date)

IV Summary and opinion

39 John is a mildly microcephalic boy with delayed speech and language development who has an abnormal relationship with his mother and has developed a reactive attachment disorder which manifests itself with his foster family to some extent and with his mother very markedly. His mother had a disturbed childhood, with alleged sexual abuse by her brothers, little perceived affection from her parents, and was early precipitated into lone parenting with no support from her family. She herself was taken to doctors an excessive amount in childhood, and this pattern has continued with at least two of her three children. It is likely that this anxiety about health pre-dated David's death but was probably enhanced by it. It was noted that the mother was not coping with David, who had several admissions, was failing to thrive and for whom respite care was requested by his mother before his early death. David's mother was seen to be rough and aggressive with him. Peter had early apnoeic attacks, three near drownings and a non-accidental injury from his mother, as well as numerous admissions and general practitioner attendances. The pattern continued with John who was subjected to admissions, investigations and inappropriate restriction of diet mainly initiated by his mother.

40 In my opinion, John has been significantly harmed by his mother's behaviour towards him, and I believe that both David and Peter similarly may have been significantly harmed.

41 I am of the opinion that Peter is lucky to have survived his infancy and that he shows signs of an anxious, constricted personality, somewhat hypochondriacal and inappropriately protective of his mother.

42 Reactive attachment disorder is a diagnostic category in the International Classification of Diseases, 10th revision. It is a constellation of social, emotional and behavioural difficulties recognised to be a probable consequence of

---

Psychiatric report: John JONES
Dr (Psychiatrist's name)

Case reference: (——)
(Date)

severe parental neglect, abuse or mishandling. A key feature is a persistently abnormal pattern of relationships with carers. The child lacks an age-appropriate interest in their primary carer and responds with a mixture of approach, avoidance and resistance to comforting. They may be observed in different social situations and may be associated with apparently indiscriminate sociability. It is more common in children with mild disabilities who are more difficult to rear, especially if the parent has poor physical or mental health, or has a personality disorder. Physical, emotional or sexual abuse of the parent as a child is highly associated.

43   It has been suggested that we may be dealing with a form of child abuse which has been entitled Munchausen's syndrome by proxy. I outline below some of the features of that syndrome.

Outline of Munchausen's syndrome by proxy

44   Factitious illness by proxy is a life endangering and sometimes fatal condition in which a parent, usually the mother, fabricates illness in a child either by inducing physical signs of illness or by deliberately misleading the physician into believing that the child is ill. The first series of cases of non-accidental poisoning were described by Rogers *et al* (1976), who recognised it as a form of child abuse.

45   Meadow (1977) named it Munchausen's syndrome by proxy, recognising its similarity to the condition in adult patients first described by Asher (1951), where illness is induced or simulated by the patient. Meadow originally described two cases, the second of which was a young boy with recurrent hypernatraemia from the age of six weeks to one year. Excess sodium chloride had been administered by his mother who had been a nurse, who it was presumed had used gastric feeding tubes and suppositories. While treatment was being planned, the boy collapsed one night with severe hypernatraemia and died. Necropsy revealed gastric erosions. Presenting

symptoms on admission were vomiting and drowsiness. He had a sodium concentration of 160–175 mmol/l.

46 Three of Rogers *et al*'s (1976) cases were of salt poisoning and two of them died. Other children were poisoned by barbiturates, opiates, phenformin and methaqualone. Subsequently cases have been described of suffocation leading to apnoea, cyanosis, cardiac arrest, cases with gastro-intestinal symptoms from laxatives, simulated haematemesis, haemoptysis and rectal bleeding, rashes, seizures, induced sepsis and fever (Samuels & Southall, 1992). Rogers *et al* (1976) concluded that marital conflict may lead to an attack on a child unduly favoured by another parent, that the relationship between the parent and child was often characterised by over-involvement and the child could become the object of intense love or hate. The child, if old enough, might collude in the administration of drugs to protect a parent and prevent separation, and the parents may find it impossible to accept responsibility for having poisoned the child.

47 Meadow (1982) described a further 19 cases and listed the warning signals. The children were usually under six years of age. Three of the mothers were themselves suffering from Munchausen's syndrome, and many of them had nursing or medical backgrounds, although they had often failed to complete their training. Most of the mothers appeared caring and loving. If they were seen by a psychiatrist they mostly emerged without a psychiatric diagnosis. Most of the children described in the literature are injured by the mother but occasionally it is the father (Makar & Squire, 1990) or another carer, as a recent case which received considerable media coverage showed. In this latter case the injuries were caused by an apparently devoted paediatric nurse (Jenkins, 1993).

48 The syndrome is thought to be rare, although it appears that the prevalence may be greater than once believed (Schreier & Libow, 1993*b*). The condition is recognised to have a poor prognosis if the child is returned to the care of a parent who continues to deny his or her part in

his or her symptoms. Of the 302 cases reported in the literature from 1981–1992, 36 (12%) had died. In a study of comorbidity associated with fabricated illness in children, Bools *et al* (1992) found that over half of the children had other illnesses fabricated by their mothers and over a quarter had a history of failure to thrive, or non-accidental injury, inappropriate medication or neglect. The same was true of 17% of their siblings. Seventy-three per cent of the sample of 56 children had been affected by at least one of these additional problems. Eleven per cent of the siblings had died in early childhood, and 39% of them had had illnesses fabricated by their mothers. It was thought that these figures were underestimates as full data were not available for 20% of the siblings (Bools *et al*, 1992).

49   It can be seen that there are many features in this case which are consistent with this diagnosis and it must be of great concern that one child has died, and another in the family (Peter) has been affected by the maternal preoccupation with his health and the experiences of neglect, and non-accidental injury. The third child, John, is showing signs of a severe psychiatric disorder, avoidant attachment, which is associated with serious personality problems in later life. He is also more delayed in speech than would be expected from his mild microcephaly and good motor development, and this raises the question of whether there has been active interference with his development. I recommend that he has a full assessment from a psychologist, to ascertain his level of functioning.

50   In my opinion this is a case of factitious illness (Munchausen's syndrome by proxy) and the mother's background helps us to understand how it arose. It is common in such cases for the mother to have experienced care only as a result of illness, and therefore for illness to be created or exaggerated in her children in order to provide vicarious attention. A recent book on the syndrome, entitled *Hurting for Love*

Psychiatric report: John JONES
Dr (Psychiatrist's name)

Case reference: (——)
(Date)

(Schreier & Libow, 1993*a*), encapsulates in its title the psychopathology of the perpetrator parent. It has been suggested to me by the mother's solicitors that her distrust of doctors arose as a result of the failure of her locum general practitioner to attend to David in his final illness. It is clear however from the documents that the mother's disturbance predated David's death, that there were serious concerns about her care of him, and it may have been that his illness was part of the syndrome and not a cause of it.

51   It is important to understand that the mother is as much a victim as are the children and that she should not be blamed for the present situation. However to protect John (and Peter), action has to be taken with which she is likely to disagree.

52   The mother made much of the clean bill of health given by the community psychiatric nurse. The latter was presumably excluding major mental illness. She would not be qualified to make a full psychiatric assessment which would include considering the mother's personality and how it affects her parenting.

53   Treatment for Munchausen's syndrome by proxy parents is available and can be effective in some cases, but an essential pre-requisite for success is an acknowledgement by the parent that they have fabricated or induced symptoms in the child. This may take some time but I have experienced such acknowledgement, made months after the child has come into care in previous cases, to a social worker working towards eventual rehabilitation. I am very doubtful whether this could happen for John within a time-scale which is realistic for him, and in my opinion it would be dangerous to return him to his mother's care at present, or for the foreseeable future. Although the subject of these court proceedings is John, I have to say that I consider Peter to have been considerably affected by the abnormal upbringing he has experienced and consideration needs to be given to his welfare by the court. It may be appropriate that he be joined to the current care proceedings so as to have the benefit of representation by a guardian ad litem.

Psychiatric report: John JONES   Case reference: (——)
Dr (Psychiatrist's name)   (Date)

Treatment for John

54   John requires and would benefit from a full psychological assessment to ascertain the pattern of his intellectual disability. He would benefit from psychotherapeutic help for his attachment disorder but this would need to be given when he is placed in a permanent home as his carers would need to be involved in the treatment. In my opinion, he should be subject of a Care Order, and in due course placed for adoption. I am of the opinion that it would not be possible to rehabilitate him to his mother within a time-scale which would not be detrimental to his further development.

Specific questions posed of me

In (local authority solicitor's) letter of (date)

55   *General care of John.* In my opinion John has been neglected at times, has been emotionally and physically abused by being subjected to unnecessary hospitalisations, examinations, investigations and restrictions as a result of his mother's actions or omissions.

56   *Is mother suffering from Munchausen's syndrome by proxy?* Yes.

57   *Is the mother capable of being treated?* Unlikely at present because she does not accept that she has injured the children.

58   *Can John be safely returned to his mother?* No. See above.

59   *What steps ought to be taken in his best interests?* Reception into care, eventual placement for adoption, psychological assessment and psychotherapy.

In (M.'s solicitor's) letter of (date)

60   *Is the pattern of referrals in both children excessive?* Yes.

61   *Could the mother's unwillingness to accept medical opinion be related to the GP's failure to attend David?* I believe that David's death enhanced his mother's anxiety, as explained above. It is a common feature in Munchausen's syndrome by proxy. In other words it helps us to understand how

the syndrome may have arisen but it does not invalidate the diagnosis or lead us to adopt other measures to protect the children. In the same way, the fact that a mother may be so ill with, say cancer, that she cannot look after her children, would not lead us to leave the children with her because the disease is not her fault.

62   *Does the mother's own history of illnesses have any bearing on her concerns for the children's health?* Yes. I have dealt with this above, and the answer to the previous question applies here too.

63   *Would the mother's history of unstable relationships and being a single parent have a bearing on her level of anxiety and the high pattern of referrals?* Yes and see above.

64   *Does the history of the children's referrals indicate they have been invented/induced by mother, given that there are many other referrals for genuinely diagnosed illnesses?* I have dealt with this above. There are few genuinely diagnosed illnesses of any consequence apart from the microcephaly and delayed speech development (which are not illnesses as such).

Guardian's letter of (date)

65   *My opinion of the mother's parenting capabilities, potential and actual, and her ability to meet John's physical and emotional needs.* Sadly the mother has long-standing and intractable parenting difficulties and in my opinion is unable to meet the needs of her children now or in the foreseeable future unless she has treatment. Even with treatment, which she is not ready for, it will take many years for her to be able safely to parent a child.

V   Summary of recommendations

66   John has suffered significant harm and is liable to suffer more significant harm if he is not removed from his mother's care and placed for adoption as soon as possible.

Psychiatric report: John JONES   Case reference: (——)
Dr (Psychiatrist's name)   (Date)

67   Peter's position should be fully considered and represented in these proceedings.

68   The mother may be capable of benefiting from treatment but only if she accepts the part she has played in John (and Peter's) problems. Such treatment is long-term, may not be successful and would not be concluded within a time span likely to be of benefit to John.

69   John needs a full intellectual assessment from a psychologist and would benefit from psychotherapy when he is permanently placed.

I declare that this statement is true to the best of my knowledge information and belief and I understand that it may be placed before the court.

(Name and qualifications)
Consultant Child Psychiatrist

References

ASHER, R. (1951) Munchausen's syndrome. *Lancet, i,* 339–341.

BOOLS, C. N., NEALE, B. A. & MEADOW, S. R. (1992) Co-morbidity associated with fabricated illness (Munchausen syndrome by proxy). *Archives of Disease in Children,* **67,** 77–79.

JENKINS, L. (1993) Judge gives Allit 13 life terms for crimes against children. *The Times,* 29 May, 3.

MAKAR, A. F. & SQUIRE, P. J. (1990) Munchausen syndrome by proxy: father as perpetrator. *Paediatrics,* **85,** 370–373.

MEADOW, R. (1977) Munchausen syndrome by proxy: The hinterland of child abuse. *Lancet, ii,* 343–345.

—— (1982) Munchausen syndrome by proxy. *Archives of Disease in Children,* **57,** 92–98.

Rogers, D., Tripp, J., Bentovim, A., *et al* (1976) Non-accidental poisoning: an extended syndrome of child abuse. *British Medical Journal, i,* 793–796.
Samuels, M. P. & Southall, D. P. (1992) Munchausen syndrome by proxy. *British Journal of Hospital Medicine,* **47,** 759–762.
Schreier, H. & Libow, J. (1993a) *Hurting for Love.* New York: Guilford Press.
—— (1993b) Munchausen syndrome by proxy: diagnosis and prevalence. *American Journal of Orthopsychiatry,* **63,** 318–321.

Appendix   List of documentation

Bundle of GP records on John.
GP correspondence (date).
GP records on Peter and correspondence.
GP records on the mother from (date) and GP correspondence.
Hospital records on the mother, John and Peter.
Various applications to the court and court orders.
Health visitor records on John.
Community health service correspondence and records on John.
School medical records and health visitor records for Peter.
Statement of Dr W., Locum Consultant Paediatrician (date)
CONI records for John.
(Social worker's name)'s report on John (date).
(Social worker's name)'s report on the Mother undated.

Compensation claim relating to head injury

June, now aged 11, suffered a severe head injury with prolonged unconsciousness, at the age of four. As well as marked physical disability she is found to have impairment of higher cerebral functions including difficulties in organising herself leading to panic and anxiety, which is not appreciated by her father and teachers as resulting from frontal lobe damage. The process of assessment and explanation led to an improvement in this understanding, in enhanced compensation for the psychological injuries and to a greater involvement of her father in her care and support.

(HEADED PAPER)

(DATE)

PSYCHIATRIC REPORT

Re: JUNE SINGER (d.o.b. — — — : now aged 11 years)

Case reference: (——)

CONTENTS

I   Introduction

1   (Name of author)

2   (Qualifications and experience, paragraph here)

3   This report was commissioned by June Singer's solicitors (name), in connection with a claim for damages arising out of the injuries she sustained when she suffered a head injury when a heavy vase fell on her. At that time she was four years old. I saw June alone and with her mother and father on (date) at my private consulting rooms when she was 11. I have read various reports from other experts and therapists instructed. I have discussed June with Mrs X., Social Worker, from the local Child and Family Psychiatric Clinic, Mrs Y., Nursing Adviser, and Dr Z., General Adult Psychiatrist. I also requested the school to fill in my standard school report form, appended.

4   The questions that I have been asked to address are:

(a) What is June's psychiatric situation now and what is it likely to be in the future?

(b) To what extent are any present or continuing problems going to impinge on her life in the future?

(c) To what extent will June require support and, if so, of what nature?

(d) I was also asked about how June views her condition and her future aspirations.

II   Brief background history

5   June is the third child of her mother and first of her father. Her parents are not currently living together and have separated and reunited on several occasions in the recent past. Her father does play a part in June's life. [Paragraph about siblings now adult]. The household thus now consists of the mother and June.

6   June's birth and early development were normal. When she was four years of age she sustained a head injury

---

which has left permanent disability. This is well set out in various reports that I have read and this report should be read in conjunction with them.

7   After recovery from her unconsciousness and the immediate effects of the injury, June's functioning at a normal junior school was in many ways better than it is now that she has transferred to secondary school. It is only now that some of her higher level cerebral functions are seen to be impaired. These affect visual memory, organisational abilities and attention span, as well as speed of cerebration and of writing. June also has a right-sided hemiparesis with balancing difficulties and lack of binocular vision. Her speech, which was dysfunctional, has improved and apart from some slight slowness and groping for words she is able to hold a normal conversation.

III   Interviews

June

8   I saw June for the most part on her own. She is an attractive, slightly plump girl with good social skills who was able to give a good account of herself. When asked what she saw as her major problems she said: "I can't do anything with my right hand and I'm not stable on my right leg but I'm better off than some of the children at school who are permanently in wheelchairs. I feel angry when I can't do something and I know it's permanent – that it won't get better."

9   I asked her what has been the most helpful thing to her and she said, "My friends sticking by me – and Mum and Dad, but my Dad can't cope. He spends time with me but not as much as I'd like". She went on to say, "I can't control my emotions. If I'm laughing I can't stop and if I'm crying I can't stop and I get hot easily and don't feel cold very much."

10   I asked her what she liked to do best and she said she liked to draw and to listen to music. She drew a picture

for me which was a cartoon dog. She says she likes to draw cartoons but is not very good at drawing anything else. I asked her about other activities and she told me that she could not swim and was sad about that. She would also like to make jewellery but it was impossible because she could not make her right hand do very much and she had a visual problem. Her depth judgement was poor and she feels dizzy if she looks down.

11   She told me that she did not like being away from her mother because she did not feel so safe with other people. "I'd like to be independent but I can't see it happening." She told me she could dress but "couldn't do laces or zips and it takes an awfully long time".

12   I asked her how she slept and she told me that on the whole she sleeps quite well but during last summer holidays she had nightmares about going mad and "morbid thoughts about an electric chair". She worries about having bad dreams. She remembers one about her mother getting shot. I said she seemed to worry quite a bit about her mother and I asked what she thought would happen to her if her mother could not look after her. She looked quite frightened and panicky and said she did not know. She did not know whether there had been any plans made if anything happened to her mother. She went on to tell me that she could not go to bed without her mother being upstairs on the same floor. She does not worry about being in the dark but if she has a babysitter she can not go to sleep until her mother comes back.

13   She told me that she worried about the future. She had the ambition to work with animals (she has four cats). "I would have loved to work with a killer whale but I know I won't be able to." She talked with some enthusiasm about her two good friends. She told me that there are times when she gets very low in her mood. I asked her if she told her mother when she felt low and she said that she did not tell her because she had enough to cope with. Once she joined an acting club but she got pushed

over so she did not return and she has been horse-riding and has trotted on her own. She was very proud of this.

14   June was aware that the reasons why she can not do certain things reside in her brain and the effect of the accident in damaging her brain. She was fairly realistic about her future but has not got a clearly formulated career plan and cannot see what the future holds for her. On the whole I found her to be in good spirits and to have a good understanding of her disabilities and to be appropriately sad about her limitations.

Information from the mother and father

15   I saw June's parents together. June's mother told me that they had tried to make a go of it on several occasions but that her husband really could not cope with June's disability, and she found that she was looking after both of them and she could not cope with that. They have a major disagreement about the activities with which June can cope, June's father thinking that she is capable of more than her mother thinks she is. June's father said that it saves a lot of argument if he does not live at home but he does come to see June once or twice each week and he tries to help with babysitting.

16   June's mother says that June panics about anything. She is particularly panicky every Monday morning when she has to go to school and at the end of every school holiday. This has been helped to some extent by some beta-blocker medication that she has been given by her general practitioner. She seems to be frightened of any new situation. She worries a lot about writing and she sometimes has difficulty in finding words. She is full of anxieties and tends to put a brave face on it to other people but lets out all her worries to her mother.

17   June's mother says that June cannot organise herself and has to be organised. She would not, for example, make use of a notebook to help with organisation. The mother's opinion is that June would forget to look at it. June's short-term memory is not good. Her periods started in

January this year and have yet to settle down. She seems to have coped with them all right. Last year they went to the local child and family psychiatric clinic and did some work as a family but "it didn't work" and they stopped attending. June's mother gave me permission to contact the clinic. I formed the impression that June's mother was coping as well as she could but that the burden of being June's major support was affecting her own well-being.

IV   School report

18   The manager of learning support in June's school filled in my standard school report on (date). June attends (Name) school and is in a small class of seven children. She is in the middle band for most subjects. Her attendance is excellent and she is thought to be of average ability, although she is above average in her music, reading and oral expression and her written productions generally. June's fine motor control is a problem due to her accident and this affects her writing and drawing as well as the presentation of her work. She is thought to be below average in her number work, craft, games, art and handwriting. Verbally she is excellent, but needs extra time to put her ideas on paper. She also has perceptual problems which cause difficulties in technology, art, geography, science and mathematics.

19   Socially June is friendly and open and gets on well with adults and her peers. She is very well behaved and polite and her mother is seen as extremely supportive and helps June to come to terms with any problems that occur by offering positive advice.

20   On the Rutter Teachers' Scale, June scored 18. The cut-off point for psychiatric disorder is nine or above. The items which are ticked as certainly applying to her are as follows:

(a) She frequently sucks her thumb and bites her nails.

(b) She tends to be fearful of new things and new situations.

(c) She is an over-particular child.

(d) She has had tears on arrival at school or has refused to come into the building this year.

21   The items which are ticked as applying somewhat are:

(a) Tends to do things on her own.

(b) Often appears miserable or unhappy, tearful or distressed.

(c) She has poor concentration and speech difficulty.

V   Psychology report

22   Mr A., Consultant Educational Psychologist, did extensive tests with June several months ago and has since visited her school. He found June to be of good–average ability as far as her verbal intelligence was concerned, although her performance in IQ tests was in the low–average range. It is unlikely that this difference could occur by chance. He identified a particular difficulty in her perceptual skills and processing speed, and he found some higher level problems in carrying out a number of sequential tasks directly or with some manipulation. She has difficulties in structuring her thoughts and organising material in order to answer questions and this affects her written work. She writes extremely slowly and, on a test of attentional skills, her functioning fell well within the impaired range. He concluded that this was an indication of a left frontal lobe impairment as were her difficulties in self-organisation and the initiation of purposeful behaviour.

23   The behavioural check-list, filled in by June's mother, shows that June has behaviours that fall into the clinical range in the clusters of: (1) withdrawn behaviour; (2) anxiety and depression; (3) social problems; and (4) attention problems.

24   This reflects closely the items in the Rutter Teachers' Questionnaire on which June scored highly. Mr A. also gave her a self-description questionnaire and it is clear that her perception of herself is of a physically-disabled girl who is poor in mathematics, is not academic and has very poor self-esteem. He draws attention to June's mother's increasing depression and anxiety and comments that this picture is commonly found in the mothers of head-injured children and of physically-disabled children.

VI   Psychiatric involvement

25   Dr Z.'s report details the problems that June's mother has had as a result of her daughters accident, which had led to her needing psychiatric treatment for a depressive disorder. Eighteen months ago, the mother's community psychiatric nurse referred the family to the local child and family psychiatric clinic where they were seen as a family by Mrs X., clinic social worker, and Mr B., child psychotherapist. At that time, June's father was living at home and some attempt was made at trying to help the family to function better. When June was seen on her own she expressed a view that her mother needed her to be dependent and also talked about her embarrassment at her mother coming into her classroom to help her with things that she felt she could do on her own. It is not clear if the staff of the clinic were aware of the complex nature of June's cognitive disabilities. They were able, to some extent, to tease out the relative contributions of June's difficulties and her mother's difficulties and the contribution made by June's father. Although June's mother terminated the sessions and has said that they "didn't work", the clinic team felt that there had been some improvement, after a few months, in the family system.

VII   Summary and opinion

26   June is a pubertal girl who is severely disabled as a result of brain damage sustained when she was four years old. She was unconscious for two weeks and has been left with a right hemiparesis, difficulties in balance, some visual problems, some intellectual deficit and difficulties in control of her emotions and temperature.

27   In particular, as she grows older, she has had more demands made on her for higher cerebral functioning and this has led to greater difficulty in organising herself, in paying attention and with memory, particularly her visual memory. On the whole, she can be well motivated but needs considerable prompting. June's verbal intelligence is average and her good verbal ability has made her more aware and insightful about her deficiencies compared to an otherwise similar person with more blunted abilities. As a result of this, she has become more anxious and somewhat depressed as she has entered puberty. She is also aware of her mother's depression and seeks to protect her mother from the full knowledge of her own unhappiness because her "mother has enough to cope with".

28   June is also sad about the break-up of her parents' marriage and feels let down by her father because he takes less interest in her than she would like. Clinically, and on standardised questionnaires, June shows evidence of an anxiety disorder which reaches phobic levels at the beginning of the school week and school term. It is greatly to the credit of her mother and the school working in concert that some of these problems are being overcome. However, in my opinion, more specific school help is needed, as recommended by Mr A. The burden of the single-handed care of June is becoming too great for her mother and it is likely that she will find her ability to cope even more impaired as June grows older. June's dreams are to do with her mother and in particular her fear of what would happen to her if anything happened to her mother. She had an experience of this when her

mother was admitted to hospital last summer and there was an increase in June's panic and anxiety.

29   In addition to a clinical anxiety disorder June suffers from very impaired self-esteem. This is of course not a psychiatric disorder but there is a high correlation between impaired self-esteem and later psychiatric disorders, including depression.

30   June would benefit at this stage from having her own counsellor with whom she could have a confidential relationship and who could help her to take a more realistic view of her achievements, which are considerable. Counselling of this kind is often available within a comprehensive school from the school counsellor. If it is not available at school it should be bought as, in my view, it would be preferable for her to receive counselling within the school than to burden her with a regular appointment to which she would have to be conveyed outside the school. It is likely that she would need sessions once every week in term time for at least one year, and subsequently at other crisis points in her life. Currently this would cost £30–40 per session. Assuming a 40-week year she will need £1600 for the first year and 10–12 sessions a year for the following six years: £3000–£4480 in total. An amount needs to be added for increases in fees. Mr A. suggests that she would also benefit from some help with organising and acquiring study skills. This would need to be organised by someone who had a good knowledge of the difficulties of frontal lobe cerebral dysfunction and I suggest that either Mr A., or one of the neuro-psychologists at Blue Children's Hospital, be consulted about this.

31   I am here recommending counselling to help June understand her difficulties and improve her self-esteem. This is separate from help with study skills. June needs an explanation from a clinical or educational psychologist who is familiar with the problems of head-injured children about the reason why she panics, why she finds it difficult to organise herself and why she finds it

difficult to control her emotions. It would be helpful if someone sat down and explained to her about the functioning of the brain and how it has come about that she has these difficulties. In my opinion this in itself would be therapeutic. It would be better if both her parents were present when this explanation is given to her so that they can reinforce her understanding. At the same time she can be told about the ways in which she can get round these difficulties and this is where the education in study skills would be appropriate.

32 The suggestions made by Mr A. and others about encouraging June's independence by a sixth-form residential college for disabled children is, I think, a good one. However, in order for June to make the best use of such a college she will need considerable one-to-one support and this may need to be reflected in the quantum of compensation. I agree with Mrs Y.'s recommendations.

33 The problem with the kinds of higher cognitive difficulties that June has is that they are not easily recognisable by even the intelligent layman and it is not surprising that her father has formed the view that she can do more than she can.

34 Mrs Singer's depression needs vigorous treatment because it is impairing her own functioning and therefore her ability to help June. June's mother and father should be encouraged to discuss the question of carers for June in the event that Mrs Singer is incapacitated. June needs to know precisely who would look after her in the unlikely event that anything happened to her parents and she needs to feel confidence in that person's ability to understand her problems.

VIII Conclusion

35 June's severe head injury has left her with significant permanent physical disabilities. She has, in addition, moderately severe higher level cognitive disability. These physical and cognitive disabilities have led to

difficulty in the development of self-esteem which in turn has influenced the development of an anxiety disorder. The increasing gap between June's abilities and her aspirations and her good insight into her disabilities is likely to lead in due course to a depressive disorder unless she can be helped to improve her self-esteem and to improve her way of dealing with her organisational and attentional difficulties. This requires urgent attention and I would recommend that she should see a clinical psychologist locally in order that she can be helped to understand more about her difficulties and the ways in which she can be helped to adapt to and overcome them.

36   June is at considerably enhanced risk of developing a depressive disorder in later adolescence or early adult life. Other possible life events which will enhance a risk further are a deterioration in her mother's health, psychosocial and psychosexual difficulties which include the possibility of single parenthood. I recommend that she receives individual confidential counselling within the school setting plus specific study skills help from someone who has a training and understanding in higher cognitive difficulties resulting from brain damage.

37   Proper arrangements need to be made for alternative carers for June with whom she can feel comfortable and confident both to relieve her mother's burden and to take over her care in the event of anything happening to her mother.

I declare that this statement is true to the best of my knowledge information and belief and I understand that it may be placed before the court.

(name and qualifications)
Consultant Child and Adolescent Psychiatrist

Appendix: List of documentation (not included here)

Glossary of legal terms used in the text

RICHARD WHITE

Editorial comment

With respect to psychiatric terminology, witnesses should expect to be asked in court to define and discuss technical words and phrases included in, or relevant to, their reports. They should be prepared at all times to provide this service.

Lawyers, on the other hand, have the task of asking the questions appropriate for the elicitation of this information. Judges and magistrates may make their own inquiries into evidence which they consider to be obscure, irrelevant, ill-defined, or contentious.

It would be inappropriate to provide here a limited glossary referring only to the few psychiatric terms included in the text. Potential witnesses are advised to prepare appropriately for the framework outlined above. For a comprehensive glossary see Gregory (1988).

Witnesses also should be prepared to explain and comment upon psychiatric diagnoses and classification systems.

Note. Unless otherwise stated, section numbers below refer to the Children Act 1989 (England and Wales).

Accommodation   the word is used in several senses. It is a service which a local authority may provide for a child under s.20, if it considers that to do so would safeguard and promote the welfare of the child. In circumstances specified in s.21, where children are removed or kept away from home, the local authority has a duty to provide accommodation. For a "child in need" (q.v.), there is a duty to provide accommodation in certain circumstances but (subject to s.20) the parent can remove the child from accommodation at will. A child who is accommodated comes within the definition in s.22(1) of being "looked after" where that accommodation is provided for more than 24 hours.

Adoption order   made by an authorised court under the Adoption Act 1976, s.12, the effect of which is to vest in the adoptor or adoptors the parental responsibility (q.v.) in relation to a child. The order operates to extinguish any parental right or duty vested in a parent or guardian immediately before making the order.

Appeal   from the magistrates' court to the High Court and from the county court and the High Court to the Court of Appeal.

Authorised person   the National Society for the Prevention of Cruelty to Children (NSPCC) and any of its officers and any person or officer of a body authorised by the Secretary of State to bring care or supervision proceedings under s.31. As at August 1996 no other person had been authorised. Persons may also be authorised for other specific statutory functions (see e.g. s.87, the inspection of independent schools).

Boarding-out   fostering of a child by an agency under the Foster Placement (Children) Regulations 1991.

Care order   an order under s.31(1)(a) placing a child in the care of a designated local authority. Unless expressly provided to the contrary it includes an interim care order under s.38.

Case law   decisions of the higher courts which establish precedent in the interpretation of statute or other subsidiary legislation or previous case law. It is binding on a lower court.

Child   by s.105(1) a person under the age of 18 years except for certain financial purposes in Schedule 1.

Child assessment order   an order under s.43.

Child in need   as defined by s.17(10).

Concurrent jurisdiction   by s.92(7) "the court", subject to any express provision, is the High Court, the county court and the magistrates' court (the family proceedings court), so that all these courts have jurisdiction under the Act.

Conditions   by s.11(7) a section 8 order may impose conditions which must be complied with by any person in whose favour the order is made or who is a parent of or has parental responsibility for the child or with whom the child is living. In relation to a child in care, a contact order may by s.34(7) impose such conditions as the court thinks fit.

Consent   one of the responsibilities of a parent in relation to, for example, the medical treatment of a child. If the child is capable of making an informed decision, his or her consent may of itself be sufficient, and it may be required, even though the court has made an order under the Children Act 1989 (see p.113).

Contact order   *either* an order under s.8 requiring the person with whom the child lives, or is to live, to allow the child to visit or stay with the person named in the order, or for that person and the child otherwise to have contact with each other, or an order under s.34 where the child is in care, requiring a local authority to permit the child to have contact with a specified person. Such an order may be subject to directions by the court.

Custody   the term used to describe the right of a parent to exercise power over a child and the order so granted in proceedings before the Children Act 1989. Legislation in which the word is used, such as the Guardianship Acts 1971 and 1973, was repealed by the Children Act 1989.

Custodianship   an order made under the Children Act 1975, s.33, repealed by the 1989 Act, vesting legal custody in one or more non-parent applicants. The order suspended the right of any other person.

Development   physical, intellectual, emotional, social or behavioural development (s.31(9)).

Directions   by s.11(7) a section 8 order may contain directions about how it is to be carried into effect. By s.38(6), where it makes an interim care or interim supervision order, the court may give such directions (if any) as it considers appropriate with regard to medical or psychiatric examination or assessment. By s.44(6), directions as to contact or medical or psychiatric examination or assessment may be made on making an emergency protection order or made or varied at any time while it is in force. By Schedule 3, a supervision order (q.v.) may contain a direction that the supervised person or the responsible person (q.v.) comply with certain directions given by the supervisor. The court may also give directions as to the conduct of the proceedings.

Directions Hearing   a brief hearing at which judge and advocates aim to decide the estimated length of the full hearing, what evidence may be agreed and what witnesses shall be called. The aim is that definitive hearings will be as effective and economical as possible.

Emergency protection order   an order under s.44 or s.45.

Ex parte   an application made to a court in an emergency, without the issue of a summons giving notice to other interested persons. This may be done to avoid informing them about the nature of the application. If others are informed of the application, it is said to be made *ex parte* on notice. An emergency protection order may be made *ex parte,* but s.45(11) specifically contemplates the possibility of such an application being made on notice.

Free for adoption, freeing order   a child in respect of whom an order under the Adoption Act 1976, s.18, has been made. The order transfers parental responsibility to the applying adoption agency, who can then place the child for adoption, so that applicants for an adoption order need not obtain parental agreement to adoption. This is not to be confused with leave to place for adoption, an order which used to be made in wardship proceedings, where the court gives its consent to the placement without dealing with the question of parental agreement.

Guardian   a testamentary guardian, a person appointed by deed, will or by the court to be the guardian of the child (s.5).

Guardian ad litem   a person appointed by the court for the purpose of specified proceedings in accordance with s.41 or for the purpose of proceedings under the Adoption Act 1976 to safeguard the interests of the child in the manner prescribed by rules of court. There is a panel of guardians ad litem comprising social workers, probation officers and other persons with appropriate qualifications.

Harm   ill-treatment or impairment of health or development (s.31).

Health   physical or mental health (s.31).

Ill-treatment   includes sexual abuse and forms of ill-treatment which are not physical (s.31(9)). By implication it includes physical abuse.

Inherent jurisdiction   the powers of the High Court to make orders in respect of the child outside the provisions of any statute. These have hitherto been exercised in the wardship jurisdiction, but s.100 of the Act limits this.

Injunction   a court order requiring a person to do something or refrain from doing something. Infringement of it is a contempt of court and punishable by fine or imprisonment (cf. prohibited steps order).

Interim care order   an order made by a court placing a child in the care of a local authority, usually pending the full hearing of an application, for a period specified by s.38(4).

Interlocutory   an order or application in the course of proceedings, that is after commencement but before final hearing.

Legal custody   so much of parental rights and duties as relate to the person of the child (including the place and manner in which his or her time is spent) (Children Act 1975, s.86). The term was used in proceedings, which have been repealed by the 1989 Act.

Looked after   defined by s.22(1) as a reference to a child who is in the care of a local authority or is provided with accommodation by an authority in the exercise of functions referred to an authority's social services committee under the Local Authority Social Services Act 1970. This includes a child subject to an emergency protection order.

Non-molestation order a term used in respect of a court order under the Family Law Act 1996 prohibiting a person from molesting an associated person or a relevant child.

Official Solicitor   his office is part of the Lord Chancellor's Department, his senior staff are solicitors and much of his investigative work is carried out by other civil servants. A substantial part of his work involves the representation of children, though he also acts for other people under disability. He acts primarily in the High Court, where he may represent children in wardship or adoption proceedings.

Occupation order a term used in respect of a court order under the Family Law Act 1996 regulating occupancy of the (matrimonial) home.

Parent   this word includes the mother and father of the child, whether or not they are or were married to each other (see s.1, Family Law Reform Act 1987).

Parental responsibility   all the rights, duties, powers, responsibilities and authority which by law a parent of a child has in relation to the child and his or her property (s.2). A mother and father of the child who were married at the time of the birth have parental responsibility. This statutory provision is extended by reference to s.1 of the Family Law Reform Act 1987 to include the mother and father of a person who is adopted or who is legitimate or legitimated (e.g. by marriage of the mother and father after the birth) in accordance with the Legitimacy Act 1976 or otherwise. The time of a person's birth includes any time during the period beginning with conception or insemination resulting in birth. In other cases the mother has parental responsibility and the father may acquire it in accordance with s.4.

Parties   persons with an interest in court proceedings who are entitled to attend the hearing, present their case and examine witnesses.

Partnership   a concept introduced in the Guidance to the Children Act 1989, in particular to reflect the working relationship between local authorities and those with parental responsibility.

Prohibited steps order   under s.8, defined as an order that no step which could be taken by a parent in meeting parental responsibility for a child, and which is of a kind specified in the order, shall be taken by any person without the consent of the court.

Putative father   a colloquial term to describe the person thought to be the father of a non-marital child.

Recovery order   an order made under s.50 by which the court can require the production of a child.

Relative   a grandparent, brother, sister, uncle or aunt, whether of the full blood or half blood or by affinity or a step-parent (s.105(1)).

Reporting officer   an officer appointed by the court in adoption proceedings, where the parent has agreed to the making of an adoption order, *inter alia* to witness the parent's agreement (see guardian ad litem).

Residence order   an order under s.8 settling the arrangements to be made as to the person with whom the child is to live. If the order is made in favour of any person who does not otherwise have parental responsibility, they acquire it by virtue of the order.

Responsible person   in relation to a supervised person, any person who has parental responsibility for the child and any other person with whom the child is living (Sch.3, para.1).

Specific issue order   an order under s.8, giving directions for the purpose of determining a specific question which has arisen, or which may arise, in connection with any aspect of parental responsibility for a child.

Supervision order   an order under s.31(1)(b) putting a child under the supervision of a designated local authority or of a probation officer. Schedule 3 contains details for the exercise of supervision orders.

Sub poena (witness summons in the magistrates' court)   court order compelling the attendance of a witness at court to give evidence. It may include the requirement to produce documents.

Voluntary care   this term was used where a child was received into care under the Child Care Act 1980, s.2. It is no longer in use.

Ward of court   a child who is under the protection of the High Court in wardship proceedings. No important step in the life of the child may be taken without the consent of the court. By s.100 of the 1989 Act, no child in care may be a ward of court. See also inherent jurisdiction.

Note on legal references

Law in the United Kingdom is based on statute, that is, Acts of Parliament, supplementary legislation, such as regulations, and rules of court. Case law is the judges' interpretation of statute and common law, the latter being a body of law built up through cases. There is a hierarchy of courts which establish precedent through decided cases. In England and Wales these courts are, in order of increasing superiority, the High Court, the Court of Appeal, and the House of Lords.

Cases which may add to the body of legal precedent are reported in the law reports, of which there are many different types. The most frequently referred to in the field of family law are the *Family Law Reports* and *Family Court Reporter*. Law reports can be found in many reference libraries and in local authority legal departments. Legal references are cited by the name of the case, the year (sometimes given in square brackets), the volume number followed by the abbreviation for the law report, and the page number.

References

ADCOCK, M., KANIUK, J. & WHITE, R. (EDS) (1993) *Exploring Openness in Adoption*. Croyden: Significant Publications.

—— & WHITE, R. (eds) (1984) *Good Enough Parenting*. London: British Agencies for Adoption and Fostering.

—— & —— (eds) (1998) *Significant Harm : Its Management and Outcome* (2nd edn). Croydon: Significant Publications.

ALDGATE, J. (1990) Foster children at school: success or failure? *Adoption and Fostering*, **14**, 38–49.

AMERICAN PSYCHIATRIC ASSOCIATION (1994) *Diagnostic and Statistical Manual of Mental Disorders* (4th edn) (DSM–IV). Washington, DC: APA.

ARBANEL, A. (1979) Shared parenting after separation and divorce: a study of joint custody. *American Journal of Orthopsychiatry*, **49**, 320–329.

BALDWIN, J., LEFF, J. & WING, J. (1976) Confidentiality of psychiatric data in medical information systems. *British Journal of Psychiatry*, **123**, 417–427.

BAZELL, C. (1989) Evidential and procedural problems in child care cases. *Journal of Family Law*, **19**, 35–38.

BENNATHAN, M. (1992) The care and education of troubled children. *Young Minds Newsletter*, **10**, 1–7.

BENTOVIM, A., ELTON, A., HILDEBRAND, J., *et al* (1988) *Child Sexual Abuse Within the Family: Assessment and Treatment*. London: John Wright/Butterworth.

BERG, I. & NURSTEN, J. (1996) (eds) *Unwillingly to School* (4th edn). London: Gaskell.

BERRIDGE, D. & CLEAVER, H. (1987) *Fostering Breakdown*. London: National Children's Bureau, Basil Blackwell.

BLACK, D., NEWMAN, M., HARRIS-HENDRIKS, J., *et al* (eds)(1997) *Psychological Trauma: A Developmental Approach*. London: Gaskell.

BOHMAN, M. (1981) The interaction of heredity and environment: some adoption studies. *Journal of Child Psychology and Psychiatry*, **22**, 195–200.

BOOTH, Mrs Justice (Chairman) (1983) *Matrimonial Causes Procedure Committee: Consultation Paper*. London: Lord Chancellor's Department.

BRANDON, S., BOAKS, J., GLASER, D., *et al* (1998) Recovered memories of childhood sexual abuse. Implications for clinical practice. *British Journal of Psychiatry*, **172**, 296–307.

BRITISH MEDICAL ASSOCIATION (1991) *Guidelines for the Access to Health Records Act (1990)*. London: BMA.

BURGOYNE, J., ORMROD, R. & RICHARDS, M. (1987) *Divorce Matters*. Harmondsworth: Penguin.

BUTLER-SLOSS, E. (1988) *Report of the Enquiry into Child Abuse in Cleveland 1987*. London: HMSO.

CHILDREN ACT ADVISORY COMMITTEE (1994–1995) *Children Act Advisory Committee Report*. London: HMSO.

CLARKE, A. M. (1981) Adoption studies and human development. *Adoption and Fostering*, **104**, 17–29.

210

COPE, R. (1995a) Mental Health Legislation. In *Seminars in Practical Forensic Psychiatry* (eds D. Chiswick & C. Cope), pp. 272–309. London: Gaskell.

—— (1995b) Civil Matters. In *Seminars in Practical Forensic Psychiatry* (eds D. Chiswick & C. Cope), pp. 310–328. London: Gaskell.

COTTRELL, D. & TUFNELL, G. (1996) Expert reports – what constitutes good practice? *Family Law*, **26**, 159–161.

CRIMINAL INJURIES COMPENSATION BOARD (1989) *Criminal Injuries Compensation to Children.* London: CICB (Now Criminal Injuries Compensation Authority).

DEPARTMENT OF HEALTH (1991a) *Working Together Under the Children Act 1989: A Guide to Arrangements for Inter-Agency Cooperation for the Protection of Children from Abuse.* London: HMSO.

—— (1991b) *Patterns and Outcomes in Child Placement. Messages from Current Research and their Implications.* London: HMSO.

—— (1994a) *The Challenge of Partnership in Child Protection: Practice Guide.* London: HMSO.

—— (1994b) *Terms and Conditions of Service of Hospital Medical and Dental Staff, July 1994.* London: HMSO.

—— (1995) *A Memorandum of Good Practice.* London: HMSO.

DEPARTMENT OF HEALTH AND SOCIAL SECURITY (1983a) *Assessments and Statements of Special Educational Needs,* HC (83) 3 LAC (83) 2. London: HMSO.

—— (1983b) *The Mental Health Act. Memorandum on Parts I to VI, VIII and X.* London: HMSO.

—— (1988a) *Working Together for the Protection of Children from Abuse,* LAC (88) 10 HC (88) 38. London: HMSO.

—— (1988b) *Working Together: A Guide to Arrangements for Inter-Agency Cooperation for the Protection of Children from Abuse.* London: HMSO.

—— (1988c) *Diagnosis of Child Sexual Abuse: Guidance for Doctors.* London: HMSO.

—— (1988d) *Guidance for the Medical Profession on the Diagnosis of Child Sexual Abuse,* PL/CMO (88) 18. London: HMSO.

FRATTER, J., ROWE, J., SAPSFORD, D., *et al* (1991) *Permanent Family Placement: A Decade of Experience.* London: British Agencies for Adoption and Fostering.

GENERAL ASSEMBLY OF THE UNITED NATIONS (1989) *Convention on the Rights of the Child.* Geneva: United Nations.

GENERAL MEDICAL COUNCIL (1987) *Professional Conduct and Discipline: Fitness to Practice.* London: GMC.

—— (1995) *Duties of a Doctor.* London: GMC.

GILL, O. & JACKSON, B. (1984) *Adoption and Race.* London: Batsford Academic.

GOLDSTEIN, J., FREUD, A. & SOLNIT, A. (1980a) *Beyond the Best Interests of the Child.* London: Burnett Books.

——, —— & —— (1980b) *Before the Best Interests of the Child.* London: Burnett Books.

GREGORY, R. L. (ed.) (1988) *The Oxford Companion to the Mind.* Oxford: Oxford University Press.

GRENVILLE, M. D. (1988) School attendance: supervision by the courts. *Journal of Family Law*, **18**, 488–491.

GROUNDS, A. (1995) The criminal justice system. In *Seminars in Practical Forensic Psychiatry* (eds D. Chiswick & C. Cope), pp. 87–105. London: Gaskell.

HARRIS, K. (1985) *Transracial Adoption: A Bibliography.* London: British Agencies for Adoption and Fostering.

HARRIS, N. (1987) Tackling truancy: the legal options. *Family Law*, **17**, 21–24.

HARRIS-HENDRIKS, J. (1993) Forensic child and adolescent psychiatry. In *Seminars in Child and Adolescent Psychiatry* (eds D. Black & D. Cottrell), pp. 233–248. London: Gaskell.

—— & FIGUEROA, J. (1995) *Black in White: Caribbean Children in the United Kingdom.* Chichester: Wiley.

HEATHERINGTON, E. M., COX, M. & COX, R. (1979) Family interaction and the social, emotional and cognitive development of children following divorce. In *The Family: Setting Priorities* (eds V. Vaughan & T. Brazelton). New York: Science and Medicine.

HERMAN, J. L. (1992) *Trauma and Recovery: From Domestic Abuse to Political Terror.* New York: Harper Collins.

HERSOV, L. (1990) The seventh Jack Tizard memorial lecture. Aspects of adoption. *Journal of Child Psychology and Psychiatry,* **31**, 493–510.

—— (1994) Adoption. In *Child and Adolescent Psychiatry: Modern Approaches* (eds M. Rutter, E. Taylor & L. Hersov). Oxford: Blackwell.

HINDMARSH, P. C. & BROOK, C. G. B. (1986) Measuring the growth of children in general practice. *Journal of Maternal and Child Health,* **11**, 196–200.

HOGGETT, B. (1990) *Mental Health Law* (3rd edn). London: Sweet and Maxwell.

ILFIELD, F. W., ILFIELD, H. Z. & ALEXANDER, J. R. (1982) Does joint custody work? *American Journal of Psychiatry,* **139**, 62.

JAMES, W. & HARRIS, C. (eds) (1994) *Inside Babylon.* London: Verso.

JENNER, S. (1992) The assessment and treatment of parenting skills and deficits: within the framework of child protection. *Association for Child Psychology and Psychiatry Review and Newsletter,* **14**, 228–233.

KEMPE, C. H. & HELFER, R. E. (1987) *The Battered Child* (4th edn). Chicago: Chicago University Press.

KIRKPATRICK, M., SMITH, M., ROY, C., *et al* (1981) Lesbian mothers and their children. *American Journal of Orthopsychiatry,* **17**, 317.

KOLLER, H., RICHARDSON, S. A. & KATZ, M. (1988) Marriage in a young adult mentally retarded population. *Journal of Mental Deficiency Research,* **32**, 93–102.

KOLVIN, I., STEINER, H., BAMFORD, F., *et al* (1988) Child sexual abuse: some principles of good practice. *British Journal of Hospital Medicine,* **39**, 54–62.

KORNER, E. (Chairman) (1984) *A Report from the Confidentiality Working Group. Steering Group on Health Services Information, NHS/DHSS.* London: HMSO.

KRISBERG, B. & SCHWARTZ, I. (1983) Rethinking juvenile justice. *Crime and Delinquency,* **24**, 33–61.

LAMBERT, L., BUIST, M., TRISELIOTIS, J., *et al* (1990) *Freeing Children for Adoption.* London: British Agencies for Adoption and Fostering.

LINDSAY, C. (1995) Alternative caretakers. In *Assessment of Parenting* (eds P. Reder & C. Lucey). London: Routledge.

LUND, M. (1984) Research on divorce and children. *Family Law,* **14**, 198–201.

MAIDMENT, S. (1984) *Child Custody and Divorce.* London: Croom Helm.

MCCARTT, H.& OHMAN PROCH, K. (1993) *Contact: Managing Visits to Children.* London: British Agencies for Adoption and Fostering.

MILLHAM, S., BULLOCK, R., HOSIE, K., *et al* (1986) *Lost in Care: The Problem of Maintaining Links Between Children in Care and their Families.* Aldershot: Gower Technical Press.

——, ——, ——, *et al* (1989) *Access Disputes in Child-Care.* Aldershot: Gower Technical Press.

MITCHELL, A. (1985) *Children in the Middle: Living Through Divorce.* London: Tavistock.

—— (1988) Children's experience of divorce. *Journal of Family Law,* **18**, 460–463.

MONTGOMERY, J. (1989) The emotional abuse of children. *Journal of Family Law,* **19**, 25–29.

MULLENDER, A. (ed.) (1991) *Open Adoption: the Philosophy and the Practice.* London: British Agencies for Adoption and Fostering.

MURCH, M. (1980) *Justice and Welfare in Divorce.* London: Sweet and Maxwell.

NOBLE, P. (1983) A case report in relation to access. *Journal of Child Psychology and Psychiatry,* **24**, 297–300.

NUECHTERLEIN, K. H. (1986) Childhood precursors of adult schizophrenia. *Journal of Child Psychology and Psychiatry,* **27**, 133–144.

OATES, M. (1984) Assessing fitness to parent. In *Taking a Stand.* London: British Agencies for Adoption and Fostering.

PARKINSON, L. (1986) *Conciliation in Separation and Divorce*. London: Croom Helm.

PEARCE, J. (1995) Consent to treatment during childhood. *British Journal of Psychiatry*, **165**, 713–716.

PYNOOS, R. S. (1992) Grief and trauma in children and adolescents. *Bereavement Care*, **11**, 2–10.

—— & ETH, S. (1986) Witness to violence: the child interview. *Journal of the American Academy of Child and Adolescent Psychiatry*, **25**, 306–319.

—— & NADER, K. (1990) Mental health disturbances in children exposed to disasters: prevention intervention strategies. In *Preventing Mental Health Disturbances In Children* (eds S. Goldston, J. Yaser, C. Heinecke, *et al*). Washington, DC: American Psychiatric Association.

REDER, P. & LUCEY, C. (eds) (1995) *Assessment of Parenting: Psychiatric and Psychological Contributions*. London: Routledge.

RICHARDSON, G. & HARRIS-HENDRIKS, J. (1996) Confidentiality, consent and the courts. In *Child and Adolescent Psychiatry: A New Century* (eds J. Harris-Hendriks & M. Black) (Occasional Paper OP33). London: Royal College of Psychiatrists.

RICHMAN, N. (1971) A behavioural screening questionnaire for use with three year old children. *Journal of Child Psychology and Psychiatry*, **12**, 5–33.

ROCHEL, J. & RYBURN, M. (1988) *Adoption Today: Change and Choice in New Zealand*. London: Heinemann Reed.

ROWE, J. (1983) *Fostering in the Eighties*. London: British Agencies for Adoption and Fostering.

——, HUNDLEBY, M. & GARNETT, L. (1989) *Child Care Now: A Survey of Placement Patterns*. London: British Agencies for Adoption and Fostering.

ROYAL COLLEGE OF PSYCHIATRISTS (1981) *Guidelines on Ethical Problems of Videotape and Other Audio-Visual Recording in Psychiatry. Report of Audio-Visual Sub-Committee*. London: Royal College of Psychiatrists.

—— (1982) Emotional abuse of children. *Bulletin of the Royal College of Psychiatrists*, **6**, 85–87.

—— (1987) Confidentiality: current concerns of child and adolescent psychiatric teams. *Bulletin of the Royal College of Psychiatrists*, **11**, 170–171.

—— (1988) Child psychiatric perspectives on the assessment and management of sexually mistreated children. *Psychiatric Bulletin*, **12**, 534–539.

—— (1990) Access to Health Records Act 1990. College Guidance. *Psychiatric Bulletin*, **16**, 114–123.

RUTTER, M., TAYLOR, E. & HERSOV, L. (eds) (1994) *Child and Adolescent Psychiatry* (3rd edn). Oxford: Blackwell Scientific.

SCHWARTZ, I., JACKSON-BEECK, M. & ANDERSON, R. (1984) The hidden system of juvenile control. *Crime and Delinquency*, **30**, 371–385.

SMITH, M. & BENTOVIM, A (1994) Sexual Abuse. In *Child and Adolescent Psychiatry: Modern Approaches* (eds M. Rutter, E. Taylor & L. Hersov). Oxford: Blackwell Scientific.

SPEIGHT, N. (1989) The emotional abuse of children: a paediatrician's view. *Journal of Family Law*, **19**, 29–33.

SPENCER, J. R. & FLIN, R. (1993) *The Evidence of Children* (2nd edn). London: Blackstone.

STEWART, G. & TUTT, N. (1988) *Children in Custody*. Aldershot: Avebury.

THORPE, J. (1993) High Court decisions on the work of the medical expert. *Association for Child Psychology and Psychiatry Review and Newsletter*, **1**, 22–24.

—— (1994) Comment. *Family Law*, **24**, 533–535.

TIZARD, B. (1987) *The Care of Young Children: Implications of Recent Research* (Thomas Coram Research Unit Occasional Paper 1). London: Thomas Coram Research Unit.

—— & PHOENIX, A. (1990) Black identity and transracial adoption. *New Community*, **15**, 427–437.

—— & —— (1993) *Black, White and of Mixed Race: Race and Racism in the Lives of Young People of Mixed Parentage*. London: Routledge.

TUFNELL, G. (1993) Psychiatric reports in child care cases: what constitutes "good practice"? *Association of Child Psychology and Psychiatry Review and Newsletter,* **15,** 219–224.

—— (ed.) (1995) Points of law. *Association of Child Psychology and Psychiatry Review and Newsletter,* **17,** 35–38.

—— & COTTRELL, D. (1995) *Expert Reports: Format in Children Cases.* London: Office of the Official Solicitor.

—— & —— (1996) Good practice for expert witness reports in Children Act cases. *Clinical Child Psychology and Psychiatry,* **13,** 365–383.

TUTT, N. (ed.) (1981) *Observation and Assessment: Report of a Working Party.* Stanmore: Department of Health and Social Security.

WALCZAK, Y. (1984) *Divorce: The Child's Point of View.* London: Harper and Row.

WALLERSTEIN, J. S. & KELLY, J. B. (1980) *Surviving the Breakup. How Children and Parents Cope with Divorce.* London: Grant McIntyre.

WEST, D. (1982) *Delinquency: Its Roots, Careers and Prospects.* London: Heinemann.

—— & FARRINGTON, A. G. (1973) *Who Becomes Delinquent?* London: Heinemann Educational.

WINNICOTT, D. (1965) *The Maturational Process and the Facilitating Environment.* London: Hogarth.

WEDGE, P. & MANTLE, G. (1991) *Sibling Groups and Social Work.* Aldershot: Avebury.

WHITE, R. (1995) Young People, Mental Health and the Law. In *Together We Stand: The Commissioning, Role and Management of Child and Adolescent Mental Health Services. NHS Health Advisory Service.* London: HMSO.

——, CARR, P. & LOWE, N. (1995) The *Children Act in Practice.* London: Butterworth.

WOLKIND, S. (1994) Legal aspects of child care. In *Child and Adolescent Psychiatry* (3rd edn) (eds M. Rutter, E. Taylor & L. Hersov). Oxford: Blackwell.

WORLD HEALTH ORGANIZATION (1992) *The Tenth Revision of the International Classification of Diseases and Related Health Problems* (ICD–10). Geneva: WHO.

YARROW, W. & KLEIN, R. P. (1980) Environmental discontinuity associated with transition from foster to adoptive homes. *International Journal of Behavioural Development,* **3,** 311–322.

YOUNG, I. (1987) Child abuse: key considerations for lawyers. *Family Law,* **17,** 376–378.

Further reading

Books and articles

AINSWORTH, M. D. S., BLEHAR, M. D., WATERS, E., *et al* (1978) *Patterns of Attachment*. New Jersey, NJ: Laurence Erlbaum.

BATTY, D. (ed.) (1987) *The Implications of AIDS for Children in Care*. London: British Agencies for Adoption and Fostering.

BLACK, D. & COTTRELL, D. (eds) (1993) *Seminars in Child and Adolescent Psychiatry*. London: Gaskell.

—— (1998) Witnessing adult's violence: the effects on children and adolescents. *Advances in Psychiatric Treatment*, **4**, 202–210.

BLOM-COOPER, R. L. (1987) *A Child in Mind. The Report of the Commission of Inquiry into the Death of Kimberley Carlile*. London: Borough of Greenwich Council.

BOHMAN, M. & SIGVARDSSON, S. (1980) Negative social heritage. *Adoption and Fostering*, **3**, 25–31.

BOOTH, DAME MARGARET (1996) *Avoiding Delay in Children Act Cases*. London: Lord Chancellor's Department.

BOWLBY, J. (1969) *Attachment*. London: Hogarth Press.

—— (1973) *Separation*. London: Basic Books.

—— (1980) *Loss*. London: Basic Books.

BRIDGE CONSULTANCY SERVICE (1991) *Sukina: An Evaluation Report of the Circumstances Leading to her Death*. London: Bridge Child Care Consultancy.

—— (1995) *Paul: A Study in Neglect*. London: Bridge Child Care Consultancy.

BROWN, G., CHADWICK, O., SHAFFER, D., *et al* (1981) A prospective study of children with head injuries: III Psychiatric sequelae. *Psychological Medicine*, **11**, 63–78.

BROWNE, K. & HERBERT, M. (1997) *Preventing Family Violence*. London: Routledge.

BROPHY, J. J. (1994) Forthcoming reforms of Irish mental health legislation. *Psychiatric Bulletin*, **18**, 100–101.

CECI, S. J. & BRUCK, M. (1995) *Jeopardy in the Courtroom: A Scientific Analysis of Children's Testimony*. Washington, DC: American Psychological Association.

DENT, R. (ed.) (1998) *Dangerous Care: Working to Protect Children*. London: Bridge Child Care Consultancy.

CHISWICK, D. & COPE, R. (1995) *Seminars in Practical Forensic Psychiatry*. London: Gaskell.

DEPARTMENT OF EDUCATION AND SCIENCE (1988) *Working Together for the Protection of Children from Abuse: Procedures Within the Education Service*. London: HMSO.

DEPARTMENT OF HEALTH AND SOCIAL SECURITY & THE WELSH OFFICE (1993) *The Mental Health Act Code of Practice*. London: HMSO.

—— (1992) *Code of Practice for the Mental Health Act (Northern Ireland)*. Belfast: HMSO.

DICKSON, B. (1989) *The Legal System of Northern Ireland*. Belfast: SLS Legal Publications.

FLIN, R. H., DAVIES, G. M. & STEVENSON, Y. (1987) Children as witnesses: psychological aspects of the English and Scottish system. *Medicine and the Law*, **6**, 275–291.

GENERAL MEDICAL COUNCIL (1993) *Professional Conduct and Discipline. Fitness to Practice.* London: GMC.

GOODYER, I. M. (1990) Annotation: recent life events and psychiatric disorder in school age children. *Journal of Child Psychology and Psychiatry*, **31**, 839–848.

—— (1990) *Life Experiences, Development and Childhood Psychopathology.* Chichester: Wiley.

GOLOMBEK, S., SPENCER, A. & RUTTER, M. (1983) Children in lesbian and single parent households: psychosexual and psychiatric appraisal. *Journal of Child Psychology and Psychiatry*, **24**, 551–572.

HARRIS-HENDRIKS, J., BLACK, M. & KAPLAN, T. (1993) *When Father Kills Mother: Guiding Children Through Trauma and Grief.* London: Routledge.

—— & —— (eds) (1996) *Child and Adolescent Psychiatry: A New Century* (Occasional Paper OP33). London: Royal College of Psychiatrists.

HESTER, M., PEARSON, C. & RADFORD, C. (1997) *Domestic Violence. A National Survey of Court Welfare and Voluntary Sector Mediation Practice.* Bristol: Policy Press.

HOLMES, J. (1993) *John Bowlby and Attachment Theory.* London: Routledge.

HOGGETT, B. (1990) *Mental Health Law.* London: Sweet and Maxwell.

INTERNATIONAL SOCIETY FOR TRAUMATIC STRESS STUDIES (1998) *Childhood Trauma Remembered: A Report on the Current Scientific Knowledge Base and its Applications.* Northbrook, IL: ISTSS.

JONES, D. P. H. (1991) Ritualism and child sexual abuse. *International Journal of Child Abuse and Neglect*, **15**, 163–170.

KENNEDY, R. (1997) *Child Abuse, Psychotherapy and the Law.* London: Free Association Press.

MALUCCIO, A., FEIN, E. & OLMSTEAD, K. A. (1986) *Permanency Planning for Children.* London: Tavistock.

MULLENDER, A. (1996) *Rethinking Domestic Violence: The Social Work and Probation Response.* London: Routledge.

MURCH, M. & HOOPER, D. (1992) *The Family Justice System.* Bristol: Family Law.

NAPIER, M. (1990*a*) The attitude of the courts to post traumatic stress disorder. *Personal and Medical Injuries Law Letter*, **5**, 28–31.

—— (1990*b*) Post traumatic stress disorder: the Zeebrugge arbitrations. *Personal and Medical Injuries Law Letter*, **5**, 37–40.

NATIONAL COUNCIL FOR FAMILY PROCEEDINGS (1997) *Cleveland Ten Years On: Child Protection, What Really Matters.* Bristol: National Council for Family Proceedings

NICOL, A. R. (ed.) (1985) *Longitudinal Studies in Child Psychology and Psychiatry.* Chichester: Wiley.

PARKES, C. M. & STEVENSON-HINDE, J. (eds) (1982) *The Place of Attachment in Human Behaviour.* London: Tavistock.

PLOTNIKOFF, J. & WOOLFSON, R. (1995) *Prosecuting Child Abuse: An Evaluation of the Government's Speedy Progress Policy.* London: Blackstone Press.

RICHARDS, M. (1991) Divorce research today. *Journal of Family Law*, **21**, 70–72.

ROYAL COLLEGE OF PSYCHIATRISTS (1996) *The Evidence of Children* (Council Report CR44). London: Royal College of Psychiatrists.

RUTHERFORD, A. (1986) *Growing Out of Crime.* Harmondsworth: Penguin.

RUTTER, M. (ed.) (1980) *Scientific Foundations of Developmental Psychiatry.* London: Heinemann.

——, QUINTON, D. & LIDDLE, C. (1982) Parenting in two generations: looking backwards and looking forwards. In *Families at Risk* (ed. N. Madge). London: Heinemann Educational.

—— & GILLER, H. (1983) *Juvenile Delinquency: Trends and Perspectives.* Harmondsworth: Penguin.

—— & SMITH, D. J. (1995) (eds) *Psychosocial Disorders in Young People.* Chichester: Wiley.

SCOTTISH HOME AND HEALTH DEPARTMENT (1990) *Mental Health (Scotland) Act 1984 Code of Practice.* Edinburgh: HMSO.

SHAW, M. (1988) *Family Placement for Children in Care: A Guide to the Literature.* London: British Agencies for Adoption and Fostering.

SHAW, R. (ed.) (1992) *Prisoners' Children: What are the Issues?* London: Routledge.

SOCIAL WORK SERVICES GROUP (1993) *Scotland's Children. Proposal for Child Care Policy and Law.* Edinburgh: HMSO.

TASKER, F. L. & GOLOMBOK, S. (1991) Children raised by lesbian mothers. *Journal of Family Law,* **22**, 184–187.

TERR, L. (1991) Childhood traumas: an outline and overview. *American Journal of Psychiatry,* **148**, 10–20.

—— (1994) *Unchained Memories.* New York: Basic Books.

TIZARD, B. (1987) *Adoption: A Second Chance.* London: Open Books.

TRISLETIOTIS, J. (1989) Foster care outcomes: a review of key research findings. *Adoption and Fostering,* **1**, 5–17.

VAN BUEREN, G. (1998) *Childhood Abused: Protecting Children Against Torture, Cruel Inhuman and Degrading Treatment and Punishment.* Aldershot: Avebury.

WALSH, E. (1998) *Working in the Family Justice System: A Guide for Professionals.* Bristol: Family Law, Jordan.

WESTCOTT, H. & JONES, J. (1997) *Perspective on the Memorandum: Policy, Practice and Research in Investigative Interviewing.* Aldershot: Arena.

WILLIAMS, R., WHITE, R., HARBOUR, A., *et al* (1996) *Safeguards for Young Minds.* London: Gaskell.

WOLFF, S. (1987) Prediction in child care. *Adoption and Fostering,* **11**, 11–17.

WOLKIND, S. N. (1979) Psychological development of the adopted child. In *Medical Aspects of Adoption and Foster Care* (ed. S. N. Wolkind). London: Heinemann.

Periodicals relevant to the field

Adoption and Fostering (quarterly). British Agencies for Adoption and Fostering, 200 Union Street, London SE1 0LX.

Childright (monthly). Children's Legal Centre, P.O. Box 3314, London N1 2WA.

Family Law (monthly). Jordan and Sons, Bristol.

International Journal of Child Abuse and Neglect (bimonthly). Pergamon Press, Oxford.

International Journal on Law and the Family (quarterly). Oxford University Press, Oxford.

Journal of the British Association for the Study and Prevention of Child Abuse and Neglect (bimonthly). BASPCAN, 10 Priory Street, York.

Journal of the Association of Child Psychology and Psychiatry (bimonthly). Academic Press, London.

Journal of the Association for Family Therapy (quarterly). Academic Press, London.

Journal of Social Welfare Law (bimonthly). Sweet and Maxwell Stevens, London.

Journal of Traumatic Stress (quarterly). Plenum Press, New York and London.

Index

Compiled by **CAROLINE SHEARD**